# TOUCHING CANCER

## MY JOURNEY OF SELF-DISCOVERY WITH ONCOLOGY MASSAGE

ELEANOR OYSTON

Foreword by Petrea King and Gayle MacDonald

First published by Ultimate World Publishing 2022
Copyright © 2022 Eleanor Oyston

ISBN

Paperback: 978-1-922828-40-8
Ebook: 978-1-922828-41-5

Eleanor Oyston has asserted her rights under the Copyright, Designs and Patents Act 1988 to be identified as the author of this work. The information in this book is based on the author's experiences and opinions. The publisher specifically disclaims responsibility for any adverse consequences which may result from use of the information contained herein. Permission to use information has been sought by the author. Any breaches will be rectified in further editions of the book.

All rights reserved. No part of this publication may be reproduced, stored in or introduced into a retrieval system, or transmitted in any form, or by any means (electronic, mechanical, photocopying, recording or otherwise) without the prior written permission of the author. Any person who does any unauthorised act in relation to this publication may be liable to criminal prosecution and civil claims for damages. Enquiries should be made through the publisher.

**Cover design:** Ultimate World Publishing
**Layout and typesetting:** Ultimate World Publishing
**Editor:** Isabelle Russell
**Cover image copyright license:** Giovanni Cancemi-Shutterstock.com

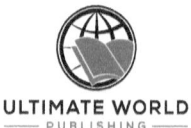

Ultimate World Publishing
Diamond Creek,
Victoria Australia 3089
www.writeabook.com.au

For Chris, Kylie, Tubi and Ian, the treasures of my heart.

# Contents

| | |
|---|---|
| Foreword | 1 |
| Note from Author | 5 |
| Introduction | 7 |
| 1. Once in a Lifetime | 11 |
| 2. The Science in a Nutshell | 29 |
| 3. The Power of Compassionate Touch | 45 |
| 4. Debunking Some Myths | 65 |
| 5. Fundamentals of Oncology Massage | 77 |
| 6. Taking OM into Hospitals | 107 |
| 7. My Heyday with OM | 127 |
| 8. Time to Move On | 147 |
| 9. OMG Is Born | 161 |
| 10. Then It Happened to Me | 175 |
| 11. Reflections | 189 |
| 12. How Can We Live Our Best Lives? | 199 |
| About the Author | 207 |
| Acronyms and Abbreviations | 209 |
| Further Reading | 211 |
| Acknowledgements | 213 |

# Foreword

Several decades ago, I confronted my own mortality as I struggled with what was meant to be a terminal prognosis of acute myeloid leukaemia. I remember well the ravages of illness and the sense of despair as I faced the prospect of leaving my two small children.

My story is a much longer tale which has been written about elsewhere, but within a couple of years of my regaining my health, AIDS had darkened our lives. At this time, in early 1985, meals for hospitalised patients with AIDS were often left outside the door.

When I heard this, it broke my heart. Having just been so sick myself, I could only imagine how awful it would feel knowing that no one wanted to touch me. It took me six months to negotiate approval for a voluntary massage program for patients with AIDS at the Sacred Heart Hospice and St Vincent's Hospital in Sydney, Australia. The administrators struggled to understand why I would want to touch people with AIDS, let alone massage them. I was dumbfounded by the lack of compassion and understanding of what it was like for people as they struggled with illness and confronted their mortality.

Fortunately, since then, massage has been recognised for the great good it does for people who are suffering from life-limiting illnesses. Now, it is recognised as a profession that requires high levels of training and expertise – and appropriate remuneration for therapists' skills and training.

This, in no small part, is due to the skills, scientific rigour, tenacity and commitment of Eleanor Oyston.

Eleanor came to the Quest for Life Centre in 2000 to work on our residential programs for people with cancer and other life-threatening illnesses. Eleanor developed a range of techniques and skills that gave people with cancer more than a sense of comfort and ease. For many participants, their symptoms either disappeared or were markedly reduced following an oncology massage treatment with Eleanor. Their anxiety levels dropped, their appetites improved, their sleep was deeper and more refreshing – and there were many individual improvements that deeply affected their quality of life in a positive, revitalising way.

Eleanor, fuelled by compassion, knowledge and a desire to make a difference in people's lives, developed and perfected many skills and techniques that she then eagerly passed on to other therapists that she trained throughout Australia and beyond.

Eleanor created nationally consistent training courses in oncology massage that are delivered in every state of Australia and New Zealand, and now in Spain and Argentina too.

Not only does Eleanor excel at inspiring other therapists to perfect the skills and techniques that she developed, but her courses steep students in a deep, broad perspective about the power of healing touch when delivered by a skilled and compassionate therapist.

In these pages, Eleanor takes you on the wonderful journey that took her from being a scientist, staring down a microscope to diagnose cancer and other diseases, to a skilled trainer of hundreds of therapists who, like her, are motivated by compassion and a desire to ease the suffering of our brothers and sisters. Despite many setbacks and challenges along the way, Eleanor's belief in the power of 'touching cancer' helped to maintain her focus on improving quality of life for people with a diagnosis or history of cancer, in the community, in hospital and at the end of life.

Every person who suffers can be comforted by healing touch. Many an intractable symptom or side effect can be eased by the skill of a well-trained massage therapist. While Eleanor was a pioneer in this healing modality, she has laid the groundwork for massage to be a staple in every hospital throughout the world.

Eleanor and I have heard many more times than we can count, 'That massage was the best thing that happened to me!'

Petrea King
N.D., D.R.M., Dip. Cl. Hyp., I.Y.T.A
Quest for Life Centre
questforlife.org.au

Eleanor Oyston is a pioneer and adventurer. Wherever she went in her career, whether looking down a microscope as a cytologist, as a biochemist for a veterinary lab in Papua New Guinea or bringing oncology massage to Australia, she broke new ground. *Touching Cancer* is a personal story of service, questioning, exploration, wisdom, passion and the search for wholeness and health. By creating an opening for others to follow, Eleanor went on a transpersonal journey on behalf of us all, not only in Australia but globally. Eleanor's driving force was to help the medical world recognise the power of gentle touch and kindness.

Giving massage to people who have cancer or are recovering from it is a very intimate action. As Eleanor writes, 'It is a two-way street, affecting not only the patient, but the practitioner.' In her later life, Eleanor was the one to sit on the patient's side of the doctor's desk. Eleanor has a potent question that she asks patients, 'What stands between you and peace today?' I've since taken that question and used it in my teaching with therapists. Today as I write this foreword, I've lost my sense of peace and am reminding myself to centre into it. Thank you, Eleanor!

I had the chance to journey with Eleanor in Australia, teaching up and down the east coast. It was a trip only for the devoted. Nearly every day for four weeks we spoke to local and national groups, taught eager massage therapists, visited hospitals, and worked with grateful clients. I wish she and I lived around the corner from one another and could meet up at the pub for a beer and a laugh. I value her as a professional, a friend and a fellow adventurer.

Gayle MacDonald
M.S., L.M.T
Author of *Medicine Hands: Massage Therapy for People with Cancer* and *Massage for the Hospital Patient and Medically Frail Client.*

# Note from Author

*Touching Cancer* is a story that emerged from my memories of countless events over many years. As such, this is not a history of oncology massage (OM) in Australia but an account of my journey with OM and what I discovered about myself along the way. Many passionate and committed people have been involved with the evolution of OM and continue to facilitate its growth. Many skilled therapists with brave hearts are not mentioned due to issues of space, but I value and admire them all. Photos are included from the archives of Oncology Massage Training, Oncology Massage Limited and Oncology Massage Global and have been published elsewhere with permission.

# Introduction

Oncology massage (OM) can be described very simply. It is a type of light touch massage that is safe and effective for people whose bodies are under stress due to illness or treatment. It is undemanding on the body, it is nurturing and it is deeply relaxing.

The medical benefits of OM are easy to summarise. Research from the United States in 2004 found that common side effects of cancer or its treatment – including pain, fatigue, anxiety, depression and nausea – improved by around 50 per cent. Even shortness of breath, memory problems, dry mouth and disturbed sleep improved significantly.[1] If this was a pill, we would all be taking it!

Even so, there is much more to OM, as it has the potential to touch deeply, express compassion and connect with suffering.

In this book, I tell the story of my involvement with OM in Australia, the science behind why it works, and why specialised training is so important for the therapists who give OM. I hope that more people will learn about this amazing therapy, which will in turn lead to better quality of life for people who have experienced the shock of a cancer diagnosis, treatment for cancer or the uncertainty of a remission.

---

[1] Barrie R Cassileth, Andrew J Vickers (2004) *Massage therapy for symptom control: outcome study at a major cancer centre.* J Pain Symptom Manage; 28(3): 244-9.

The book is also about me! OM has been integral to my life over the past 20 years. I would not have been able to achieve what I have without the transformation that motivated me to adapt my mind, open my heart and use my skills in a completely different way.

Everything I did before OM led up to *that* moment when I realised the power of compassionate touch and decided that I wanted to share it with as many people as possible. For me, this meant doing something big. What happened to me over the next two decades was the steepest learning curve you can imagine. Success, failure, rejection, heart-warming connections and an absolute rollercoaster of emotions.

I didn't plan the journey; I lived it. It was all new thinking. My point of difference is that I came to this as a scientist, trained to evaluate and analyse, and my aim has been to apply those principles within the less scientific realm into which I leapt headfirst 20 years ago.

Starting OM in Australia has been my life's work, my passion, and it also cracked me wide open. When I began, the prevailing dogma was that people with cancer should not receive massage therapy. Helping to debunk that myth was the first of many challenges along the way to developing an effective technique and a nationally consistent training program, as well as attempting to respectfully integrate OM into a health system focused on treatment and quantity rather than quality of life.

The training program is taught in Australia and New Zealand and is recognised by major massage associations and the international body, The Society for Oncology Massage (S4OM) in the US. The Australian program is also being taught in Spain and Argentina.

Of course, OM will not 'fix' cancer. What it can do, however, is pave the way for greater self-care that rekindles self-awareness at the deepest level, promoting a sense of wholeness to counter the chaos and fear brought on by cancer diagnosis and treatment. OM creates a space where peace and stillness can bloom and grow.

## Introduction

Petrea King's words ring in my ears as I write this. I worked alongside Petrea on cancer programs over nine years and developed the first OM program while working at her centre, Quest for Life (QFL), in Bundanoon, NSW. Sometimes I do not know where Petrea's words start and end in my 'molecules of emotion'. I can never thank her enough for allowing me to find my own wisdom in the midst of chaos, and to find the courage to develop OM in Australia.

My career as an OM therapist and teacher has been full of laughter and tears, so it feels right to share this story here.

> It was the first day that the Austin Hospital in Melbourne allowed my OM trainee therapists into the palliative care ward. I gathered the curtains around each bed in a room where four women were in the last days of life and asked them one by one if we could give a gentle massage. All four agreed, so we retreated to the nurses' station to review files, current pathology and timing of pain relief. Together, we made a treatment plan of OM techniques. We returned to the bedsides and I watched the massages begin.
>
> The first lady was very fragile, and a brief 10-minute massage was our plan. At the end of the 10 minutes, I stepped inside the curtain in time to see the patient look into the therapist's eyes and say, 'Maybe I can die having a massage'?
>
> As the student and I left the room, four young doctors who were waiting to see the patient saw the tears in our eyes and asked if we were all right. I responded by apologising for keeping them waiting. Their response was, 'No, what you do is much more important than what we can offer.' An unsolicited affirmation that I have carried in my heart ever since.

TOUCHING CANCER

This is the story of my journey with OM and what I discovered about myself along the way. My hope is that this book inspires others to seek out information that will help them to become aware of their true nature and find ways to live their best lives.

# 1.

# Once in a Lifetime

My career has been a meandering journey, made up of decisions taken for good reasons (and often for the good of other people), that led to many changes in direction. But it all brought me to that one moment, when I first arrived at QFL in Bundanoon, while on the radio Anthony Warlow sang about a girl knowing that destiny was calling her. I was that girl!

But let's go back to the beginning.

> I was born in Scotland on a cold October night, in my parents' bed. World War II separated me from my siblings, who were ten and eight when I was born. My mum didn't want the local midwife to deliver me. My dad went to fetch the doctor, but he had an inflamed appendix, so his brother, also a doctor, had come from Edinburgh to run his practice until he recovered.

The story goes that Mum endured a long and painful labour and, in the early hours of 8 October 1948, she safely delivered a healthy 10-pound 6-ounce wee girl – me!

I was born 'face first' and if the replacement doctor, who was the professor of gynaecology and obstetrics from Edinburgh University, had not been there, both Mum and I would have surely died.

What I made of my birth story is that the universe conspired to ensure my safe arrival into this world for a reason. I am meant to be here. As I look back over my life, maybe oncology massage is the 'reason'?

In 1952, my family emigrated to Australia, and I grew up in Western Sydney, but that's another story…

## The scientist in me

I spent 25 years working in medical pathology laboratories, 15 of those diagnosing cancer in cytology and 10 years in a neuroscience research laboratory.

In 1966, aged 17, I studied medical technology at Sydney Technical College (now University of Technology Sydney). My first employer was the haematology department at St Vincent's Hospital, Darlinghurst. These were exciting times in medical science, with the first bone marrow transplants and heart transplants being performed. There were few women in the field, and we were only 'supposed' to work until we married and had children. That was never going to be me, I loved my work and was determined to have it all!

Once in a Lifetime

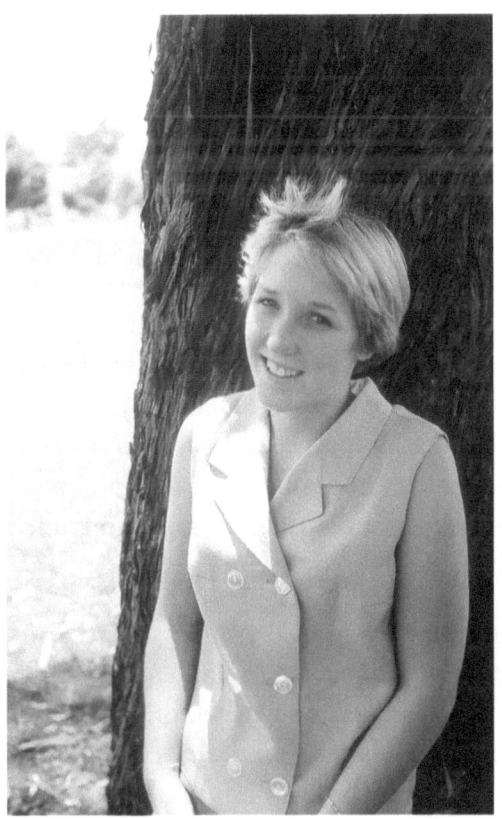

Honeymoon 1968

In 1968, I married Chris, a budding naval man, and, 52 years later, he claims credit for my amazing CV. Moving home, state and country often over the years, I became skilled at setting up house, settling children into school and finding a job.

When we moved from Sydney to Perth in 1975, I worked for Ramsey Surgical and demonstrated the new vacuum blood collection system to all of the local hospitals. It was a great way to get to know the town, understand the culture and show off my skills.

Kings Park Medical Lab then snapped me up and for the next three years I worked full-time in haematology, studied cytology in my spare time, supported my husband through a series of promotions and parented two little girls.

As I finished my studies, I was asked to join the first professor of cytology in Australia at the King Edward Hospital for Women. Another exciting and ground-breaking year followed, as cytology was growing rapidly, and the professor was generous with his time and talent.

In the 1970s, cytology was 'by hand and by eye', often without fume hoods. Automation was spoken about, although there was strong resistance as it would come at the expense of jobs. Immunochemistry was developing alongside fine needle aspiration (FNA) biopsies. I loved microscopy and sitting for hours each day at a microscope was an adventure. Every sample was different, and I often felt like Sherlock Holmes on the path of discovery.

It was while we were living in Perth that I first heard Dr Elizabeth Kubler-Ross speaking about cancer and end of life. She spoke to my heart, and I felt she understood the emotions of diagnosing cancer and of being the eyes that first saw the cancer cells that would change a life forever. I realised that I was not alone – there were doctors and scientists in my 'tribe', and my job was to find them.

> In 1978, I applied to study speech pathology. I was one of only six candidates who made it through to the last interview, then I was asked, 'If your husband is posted, will you leave the course?' I was being asked to choose between my marriage and my career. I chose my marriage. This would never happen in 2022 – or would it? I applied for university entrance four times over the years and got accepted each time only to leave the country, the state or the city because of a posting. Ah, the military life for me!

In 1979, we moved to beautiful Papua New Guinea (PNG). Running the biochemistry and haematology sections of the Veterinary Laboratory in Port Moresby was a welcome respite from diagnostic cytology and it was a great adventure.

This job gave me the opportunity to fly to places like Manus Island, Wewak and Goroka, collecting blood from Department of Primary Industry livestock. In Wewak, I tail-bled buffalo imported from the Northern Territory, in the highlands I bled goats and on Manus Island I bled dogs and chickens, looking for viruses from Asia. I learnt to scuba dive and, when my job took me to Lae and Madang, Chris came too, and we explored coral reefs together.

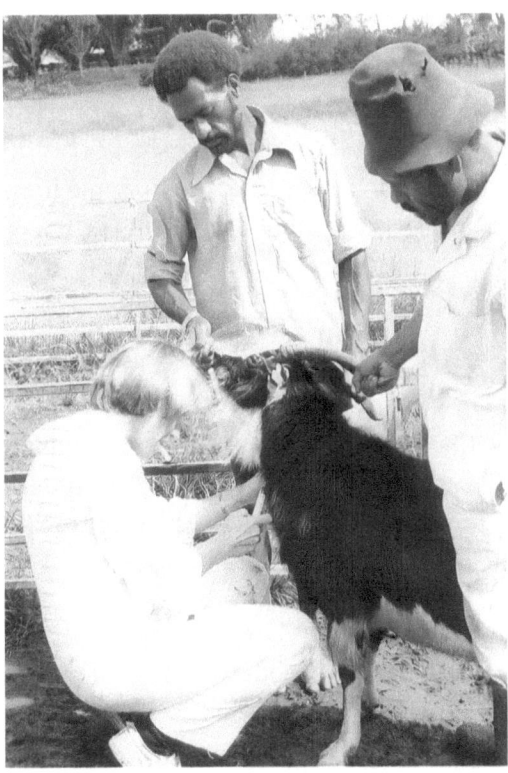

Blood collection in the field c1979

In PNG, I began to notice the power of touch. When I shook hands with an Indigenous person, they usually held my hand for quite a while. While it felt odd at first, over time I grew to deeply value this connection. At that time, most educated women in PNG did not enjoy support – they brought home the pay-packet, cared for the family and sat below their husbands socially. A handshake was often the only way I could convey my encouragement or support – gentle, safe touch.

In PNG, I met Maria von Trapp – yes, from the famous *The Sound of Music* family! Maria, the daughter of Captain von Trapp, was a missionary and she taught music in her home. Once a week, my girls had lessons after school and I slept in a comfy chair, recovering from my workday. As we were leaving PNG, Maria came to the airport to bid us farewell. She stood with our PNG national friends at the 12-foot cyclone wire fence (PNG nationals were not allowed into the airport unless they were flying) and had a friend pass a book over to me – *Something More* by Catherine Marshall. This book kindled a faith in me that has lasted a lifetime, teaching me important lessons about patience and God's timing.

### Settling in Canberra

Arriving in Canberra in July 1981 was an encounter with cold. Canberra felt like a 'grey' town. Grey buildings with grey people streaming out at close of business. No betel nut streaks down car doors, no smiling faces with bright red teeth and no noise blaring from 'boy-busses' as they chugged along.

Our two-year posting to Navy Office became 31 years in Canberra, and this beautiful city has become rather cosmopolitan for a 'big country town'.

Canberra brought us all a fantastic lifestyle, as well as job satisfaction. After a few years back in cytology at The Canberra Hospital (Woden Hospital during my time there) I took a job at the prestigious John

Curtin School of Medical Research (JCSMR) in a developmental neuroscience laboratory.

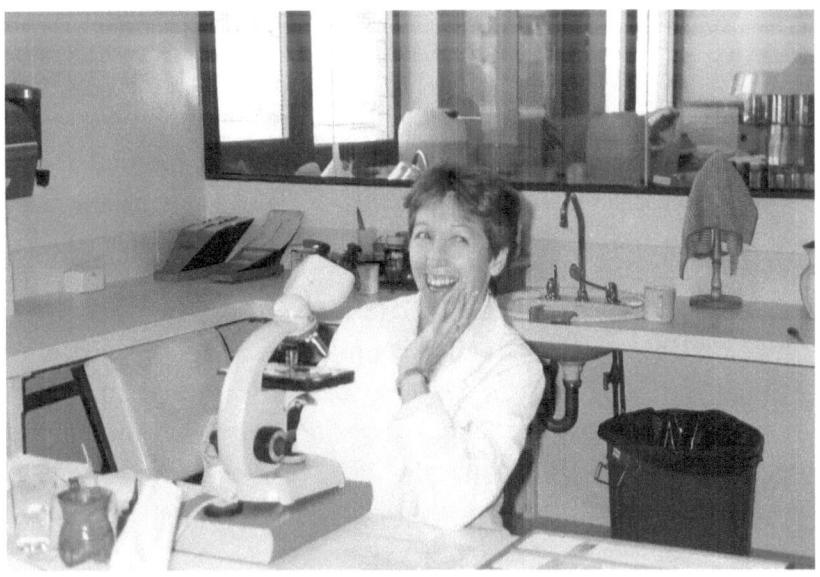

Finding humour in a stressful workplace.

A powerful influence on me at this time was Dr Caryl Hill, the senior researcher in the JCSMR lab. Caryl was determined, inventive, diligent, strong (physically and emotionally), very clever and didn't suffer fools gladly. She made her life happen, whatever it took. Caryl stayed open-minded in the face of dogma, she hosted great dinner parties and I admired her zest for life.

After four years, Chris and I adopted our son Ian from South Korea. At the time my choice had been to start a PhD or expand my family. I knew deep down that another child was more important. I had always imagined having at least four children, but Mother Nature did not agree.

I went back to cytology part-time and, when Ian was older, I returned to work at JCSMR. I remember this time as very busy. The lab work was very flexible and even with a lot of responsibility, I was trusted to work from home if needed. Adding to the busy work and family life, we were very active in the Uniting Church.

## Looking beyond the lab

After 10 years in medical research, I wanted a change from test tubes, harsh chemicals and long hours. I took on a health education degree at the University of Canberra, paid for by JCSMR, with an afternoon a week off to attend lectures.

This course focused on our health and research systems, the World Bank, Big Pharma and other heart-numbing topics. The degree included six months of sociology and I attended every class with gritted teeth. I found the world of economics shocking. The readings supplied by the lecturers began to give me a language through which I could share my awakenings or 'knowing' about the world of science I had joined straight from school.

I was a good lab technician. I had been taught well and had seen a lot of my excellent work slipped into the bottom drawer because we were 'too far ahead' to get funding for the project. Monoclonal antibodies and *in situ* hybridisation science were at the cutting edge of my work so I was well placed to use all my skills of hospital-based histology, frozen section techniques and tissue culture. I knew that collaborative research depended on the personality of the researcher, the level of scientific status that accompanied a breakthrough and who received recognition, as well as the funding that might be 'floating' around. I ultimately became disillusioned with the politics.

Is that what makes a middle-aged scientist jump off the cliff of a steady, safe, socially acceptable career and dive headfirst into the murky world of complementary therapies? It wasn't quite that simple!

Feeling like I was 'meant' to be on Planet Earth has had consequences. I have never resisted walking down new paths, going on adventures or exploring ideas.

When I left the research lab in 1997, I started work as an occupational rehabilitation consultant at the behest of a friend looking for staff for his business. When we began the conversation, I did not know what a rehabilitation business was, yet three weeks later I was a consultant! However, I did know how every cell in the body worked, how pain medication worked, how to support gut health and I could write an accurate report.

I worked on billable minutes, had 30-plus clients for major insurance firms and thought the job was about helping folk get back to work in a safe and supportive workplace. I was very naïve, and thank goodness I was a fast learner. I clearly saw the positive outcomes for people with musculoskeletal injuries when I found them a skilled and confident massage therapist.

After three years, I was burnt out, disillusioned once again and in dire need of a holiday.

### Discovering a new me in Africa

The year I turned 50, I wanted to climb Mount Kilimanjaro. Every time I spoke about my dream, a friend or family member said, 'I'll come.' I quickly realised that I wanted to 'go it alone'. Encouraged by Chris, I bought return flights to Johannesburg and planned a month in South Africa all by myself. Kilimanjaro was not possible as I was not vaccinated for that part of Africa, but it was an adventure all the same. Visiting game parks, hiking in the Drakensberg Mountains, catching up with colleagues from PNG and so much more.

I came home from my holiday knowing again that, in the wise words of Petrea King, something had to change, and it was me. I had taken off all my 'labels' – wife, mother, daughter, sister and even friend. I was a free spirit for the first time in my life and I realised that I really liked *me*!

It became clear that I was ready to do something completely new. I had been immersed in science, started teetering on the edge of an evolving world, and I knew in my soul that there was much more to see and know.

## Going to massage school

Why did I study massage? To start with, because it worked in with my life and gave me time to prioritise my family. I stumbled on massage training by accident, but it became the key to my future.

I worked as a remedial massage therapist for 12 months after massage school, doing eight to ten massages a day at the age of 53. I realised that deep tissue and trigger point work was not sustainable, so I investigated Bowen therapy (BT) with its basis in fascial release, which is gentle on the client and therapist alike and offers great results for both injury and emotional release.

The week after I finished my diploma at massage school, I started teaching pathophysiology to massage students. I was told that it was the first pathology course in Australia in 2001. The course involved 10 three-hour lectures. I had over 30 years of science in my head, which was very difficult to condense!

I wrote and published the course, then taught it for three years. Each year I learned more about the gaps in therapists' understanding of the body and disease processes. Apart from nurses or other health professionals looking for a change, many of the people I met at massage school were kind-hearted folk who had learned little or no science. I discovered first-hand what therapists need to know about systemic diseases like diabetes, heart disease and cancer. This was a time when massage schools were teaching students not to touch sick clients, to send them away as 'untouchable'.

It was not long before I used all this experience in my work at QFL.

## Taking it all to QFL

I met Petrea King in 1998, shortly after I began my stint as a rehabilitation consultant. Different insurance companies referred clients with back injuries, who tended to be in everyone's too hard basket. I noticed many similarities in the stories of people with 'bad backs', mostly the issues of living with chronic pain and a much-reduced income. I imagined that I could bring them together for mutual support, so I went to the QFL course on 'How to Manage a Group'. However, the insurance companies didn't like my idea, so I never got the chance to try it.

A year or so after the course, I called Petrea for advice on how to help a friend who had been diagnosed with leukaemia. Petrea asked me what I was doing, and I told her that I was 'rubbing bums' – that is, working as a qualified remedial massage therapist and a Bowen therapist! Petrea asked me if I'd like to come and massage folk at QFL.

It started as weekend work when there were enough participants to run a program. It was not about planning; it was all about 'trusting'. Petrea might ring me on Thursday to arrive in Bundanoon on Friday or she might not ring until I only had two hours to get to Bundanoon for the staff briefing. I loved the spontaneous and trusting nature of everyone on the team.

I signed up to be the massage therapist on the programs to earn some extra money. Little did I know that over the next few years, working on cancer programs with Petrea and her partner Wendie, I would experience more emotional and spiritual changes than at any point in my life to date. At QFL, I found a 'tribe' who kept my feet on the ground and my heart pounding with possibilities.

The instruction for the massage therapist at QFL was: 'Be gentle'. Petrea had a lot of experience massaging folk with AIDS and cancer and her door was always open to her team. At that time, massaging very ill people went against the prevailing and inaccurate dogma that it was not safe. Petrea's co-facilitator at the time was also an experienced massage therapist. I was the new 'kid' and found myself in the perfect place to explore my massage techniques, safe 'do no harm' touch and the power of compassionate acceptance.

Some massage therapists in these programs shied away from 'touching cancer'. They had never been taught the science of cancer or cancer treatment. I often coached therapists before and after they massaged the very sick folk on the QFL program, to allay their fears or to suggest a reason for the tactile experiences they described.

## From Massage, Cancer and More to Oncology Massage Training

After this ad hoc coaching had gone on for a while, Petrea's co-facilitator and I began talking about training therapists to massage people with cancer and, after attending an Australian Traditional Medicine Society (ATMS) conference in 2001, realised that there was a need for such a program.

The name for the new program was *Massage, Cancer and More* (MC&M). I ran the first five-day course with 12 therapists at QFL in early 2002. Generosity and compassion, laughter and tears were the impetus for developing MC&M and oncology massage training (OMT) grew organically from this simple start.

## Bringing OM to Australia

The early training programs were so successful that I started thinking about taking OM further. What I had learned from others about meditation and stillness, therapist self-care and communication were invaluable, but I wanted to begin with cell science.

I learned what was happening in oncology massage in the US and United Kingdom (UK), and the world of medically based, scientifically grounded massage techniques and research. I read books by Gayle MacDonald and Tracy Walton and I wanted to bring the groundbreaking work they were doing to Australia.

I knew that if OM was to ever be accepted by the medical profession, it had to be scientifically plausible even in the absence of a strong evidence base. Training needed to be consistent, backed by research and definitely not stray into the murky territory of pseudoscience. I kept looking with a scientist's eye and this helped to make oncology massage in Australia successful.

Could massage be respectfully integrated into mainstream medicine? That 'face first' baby was not going to take 'no' for an answer!

## Building OM as a business

I spent hours developing easy-to-understand cell science, ran the advertising portfolio, booked the venues, collected fees and ran a registry to record student exam results. I learnt computer skills to create and print certificates and sent documents via email (this was all new technology back then).

During the courses, I briefed the students, bought and made morning and afternoon teas, taught the course content and supervised the practical sessions. It was often tricky to find patients with cancer for the students to massage. This was the final segment of the course, and by then I was exhausted! There was nothing I could or would not do. Petrea would say 'you do what it takes' when you follow your passion.

By 2005, I was knocking on massage school doors asking if I could speak to their graduating students – 'Let me tell them that they cannot massage folk with cancer or a history of cancer unless they have done specific training, read the right textbooks and understand that they can do harm.' As course numbers grew, I knew I could not keep doing it by myself.

I began identifying teachers and my idea was to train and mentor a teacher in each state, focusing on the special skills needed to teach OM. Teaching OM to adult students is challenging. We are not filling up an empty vessel, we are trying to reshape thinking, including long-held beliefs that are often based on the loss or suffering of a loved one. Most of the therapists were earning a good living offering remedial massage, giving clients what they asked for – deep work, a product of the 'no-pain, no-gain' belief system. Could they earn a living through OM?

I set very high standards for my teachers. They all needed to have 'train the trainer' certification and, when I could afford it, I paid for advanced courses, overseas teaching and a robust (for its time) teaching income. I could never guarantee work, but what the program gathered in student fees, I intended to share fairly.

## David and Goliath: Moving into hospitals

In 2008, my attention turned to hospitals and the dream of training OM therapists to work alongside health professionals caring for patients with cancer, as happens in the US and UK. Cancer treatment is a gigantic structure within our medical system. What made an aging massage therapist think that she could infiltrate the inner chambers of hospitals? Sheer pig-headedness, my husband would say!

Moving my program into the integrative complementary medicine world of hospitals was huge, costly and exciting beyond anything I could have imagined. It has happened, albeit slowly. Today, oncology massage services are becoming more common in hospitals around Australia, although sustaining the services is challenging.

In 2009, I developed OMT Modules 3 and 4 and approached a large cancer hospital in Sydney to take me on. In October 2010, when the Olivia Newton-John Cancer Wellness & Research Centre (ONJCWRC) was still a hole in the ground, I was contacted to see if my courses would fit into their model. I fronted an ethics committee at the Austin Health campus, seeking approval for my in-hospital training programs. Olivia herself embraced me after I demonstrated massage at the opening of the centre just a year later.

The main hurdle for me over the past 21 years has been money, or rather, the lack of it! Running the courses is expensive, massage is a poorly paid, mostly female industry and I discovered 'small business myths'. Hospitals think I made money out of the programs I taught on their premises! Ha… ask my only benefactor, Chris Oyston. Our superannuation and his Navy pension have financed my work all this time – even this book.

How much we are prepared to pay for kindness and compassionate touch is the challenge that every hospital, university and private clinic I have spoken to grapples with as the first barrier. I notice that when money is needed by the 'right person' or 'idea' it is found. Unfortunately, power and influence tend to outweigh research results.

I have been told that a massage service is unaffordable. Science and medicine know that human touch is essential for life itself and yet compassionate touch for very sick people is prohibitively expensive! I weep.

I cannot believe how hard I worked to keep my little business going and growing. So did the others who joined me, sharing my vision of improving quality of life for people with cancer. At the best of times, we were an unassailable team, bonded through passion and persistence, bringing knowledge to therapists and comfort to clients.

By 2012, we were teaching all over Australia and in New Zealand, with a rapidly growing database of recognised therapists and some hospital positions opening up. We even developed an Australian

Skills Quality Authority (ASQA) accredited course, with five years to establish a Registered Training Organisation (RTO) to deliver the program. Sadly, my business could never afford the cost of bringing accreditation to fruition.

By 2013, OMT was a registered charity called Oncology Massage Limited (OML) that was well established nationally and internationally, and I thought I wanted to 'retire'. I began taking long holidays with Chris and watched as the new OML leadership team evolved. While travelling, I realised that Australian OM was well ahead of other countries for a variety of reasons, so when my Spanish friend asked if I could take OM to Spain, I enthusiastically agreed. Characteristically, another spur of the moment decision led to the creation of Oncology Massage Global (OMG) in 2017 and the start of a whole new adventure.

Online learning for tactile modalities was not offered in Australia back then, although it is now, as a result of the restrictions of COVID-19. Through OMG, I have developed an online Spanish program that is running in Argentina after its launch in Barcelona, Spain. Our goal for 2023 is to create an English version.

### Then it happened to me too

One in two people over the age of 75 will be diagnosed with cancer, a life-changing disease, at least once in their lifetime (ABS). This is truly a shocking statistic. As I approach my 73rd year of life, my experience and that of my peers testify to the truth of that statistic! Mercifully, Australia has an excellent medical system and a high standard of living. Due to advances in early detection technology, people with cancer in the 21$^{st}$ century are enjoying survival rates previously unheard of or even thought possible.

In 2020, I was diagnosed with multiple myeloma. You can read more about this in Chapter 10, because all I'll say here is that I'm a 'work in progress'. I actually don't know who I am right now or what I want for my future. What I do know is that I need to tell the story of oncology massage in Australia.

I hope this book raises awareness in the medical world, particularly for those involved in cancer diagnosis and treatment, to recognise the power of gentle touch, compassion and kindness.

> After about five years of working away from home for two weeks out of four during her programs, Petrea invited Chris to join the team as the senior support person. We laugh remembering that Chris was the best vomit bowl holder ever. He has a cast-iron stomach. Chris could fix any oxygen cylinder that malfunctioned and got everyone to meals on time with naval precision.
>
> Early in Chris' time on the team, I remember going to the local pub to watch the State of Origin match. This was not usual on the programs, but we had a largish group of young men who were watching their wives slowly die. The game ended, I called 'last drinks' and prepared to leave when a young dad asked me how to tell his daughters that their mum had died. I had experience with this type of conversation, yet everyone is unique. Chris listened, we 'chewed the fat', I cried with my pub mate, and we wandered back to Quest in the moonlight.
>
> When Chris and I were alone, he said, 'Now I get it, now I know why you keep coming back to Quest and why oncology massage is so important. That young man would never have had that conversation in the retreat centre, and you made him feel relaxed in the pub. He could ask the hard questions.' I'll take that as a job well done!

# 2.

# The Science in a Nutshell

Books about massage do not generally have chapters on science, but it's important to address it here. Science is critical to the story of OM because OM is based on science. An effective OM treatment requires massage therapists to know about how healthy cells and cancer cells differ, the importance of our immune systems and the role of the mind-body connection in promoting wellbeing.

I make some broad generalisations in this chapter, just as I do elsewhere in this book. In many areas, there are no double-blind research studies available, as there are with most medical treatments. This chapter is a combination of my reading of the scientific research and of my observational research, over the past 20 years. It briefly covers areas about which there are already entire shelves full of textbooks, and I encourage you to seek out more information about any area that sparks your interest. You can find a list of further reading at the end of the book.

## It all starts with our cells

Our cells are fundamental to everything that happens in our bodies. Each of our 30 trillion clever cells performs a very specific task, day in and day out, to keep our bodies functioning optimally. Normal cells behave in predictable ways. Every cell has a programmed life cycle and cells die naturally in a process called *apoptosis*.

The anchor points in a cell are called *desmosomes* – filaments of protein that help healthy cells make strong attachments to neighbouring cells, to create a functioning organ. Different body areas or organs are segmented by a *basement membrane*, a natural 'curtain', like the one separating the skin from the tissue beneath. In this way, cells stay where they are supposed to be, doing their jobs until they die and are replaced, all in a natural pre-programmed way.

A great deal of information about the body can be seen through a microscope. Assessing cytology specimens, field by field, at 400x magnification, is a painstaking process and it feels like a treasure hunt. A good cytotechnician knows what every cell in the body looks like, how infection and disease change cell structure and if we are looking at 'artefact' (changes that are caused by collecting and staining the specimen).

## What is different about cancer cells?

Diseases like cancer begin in cells that take on a range of different characteristics, sometimes quickly but mostly over many years. The changes allow the cells to evade the normal checks and controls by our immune system and stop the natural cell cycle from proceeding.

Cancer cells, to me, appeared like 'naughty children' able to get more than their share of food and attention – wilful cells that refuse to obey the rules. By nature, most cancer cells are fragile. They forget to switch off and so they keep growing and spreading. As they grow more quickly than normal cells, they do not develop strong attachment points with their neighbours, and instead, they are quick to allow chemicals and nutrients to pass through their cell walls. At this stage, the abnormal cells are still confined to one place in the body, in what is called an *in-situ lesion*.

As well as weak desmosomes, cancer cells often secrete enzymes that degrade the cell wall and allow them to pass through the basement membrane and spread directly into the adjoining tissue or through the body via the bloodstream or lymphatic system. This can lead to *metastasis*, the formation of a new growth of the same tumour in a different part of the body. We can host more than one kind of cancer cell at any given time which can make treatment very complex.

## What are the body's defence systems?

Generally, when something goes wrong in the body, our immune system comes to the rescue. Immune system cells travel in the bloodstream, searching for a signal that an area of the body needs their support. When the message is received, immune cells pass through the blood vessel wall and move through the fascia – loose connective tissue, comprised mainly of collagen and elastin, like a giant web holding all our muscles and organs in place (discussed further in Chapter 3).

When the immune cells find their target, they send for reinforcements. Some of the gathering immune cells begin to absorb abnormal proteins or damaged cells (such as cancer cells), decluttering as best they can so that the healthy immune cells and tissue cells nearby can continue their normal function. Every cell does its best to contain the problem. Our immune cells are our best friends.

Another powerful defence we have is our lymphatic system, which is like our disposal and recycling system. It is made up of lymph nodes and complex watersheds which are found in every part of the body. Lymph nodes are in larger numbers in the armpits, groin, neck, throat and abdomen. Lymph is a clear fluid that is part of the interstitial fluid that surrounds all our cells and is squeezed out of and reabsorbed by tiny blood vessels (capillaries). Excess fluid that is not reabsorbed goes into the lymph vessels. The lymph fluid eventually empties into the circulation and is disposed of by the kidneys. Once a cancer cell gets into the subcutaneous tissue (below the skin), it is the job of the lymph nodes to stop it from going any further. The cells in the lymph nodes are clever and adaptive; they watch out for pathogens of any kind (like bacteria or viruses) and any cell that is in the wrong place at the wrong time.

Of course, we hate the thought of having even one cancer cell in our bodies, but the reality is that our bodies contain trillions of cells and some of these are always cancer cells. Most of the time, when our immune system notices the cancer cells, it eliminates them before they replicate and become a problem. It is when our immune system 'falls asleep' for some reason that cancer cells have the chance to grow unchecked until some symptoms prompt further investigation.

## Cell receptors and the interstitial sea

To understand how cancer cells can take hold in our bodies, we need to go back to how cells function and examine the vital role of receptors on the cell wall. The cell receptor theory challenges a long-held belief about our cells and DNA, that genes alone determine the character and quality of our lives and that we are powerless to change our heredity.

Human Genome Project scientists working to unravel the human genetic code expected to find over 100,000 genes. However, when this long-awaited and miraculous project had been completed, the final gene count was in fact 23,000, only a couple of thousand more than insect DNA!

So, where do we get all our fine-tuning, like our capacity to learn and change in response to our environment and age, and all of the many attributes that set us apart from other species in the animal kingdom?

## The Science in a Nutshell

Pioneering work by Dr Bruce Lipton in the US led to the discovery of epigenetics (literally, 'above the genes').[2] The nucleus of the cell, the part that contains our DNA, is not the brain of the cell as we thought 40 years ago – it is the 'gonads', the reproductive blueprint that is passed from one generation to the next. The nucleus is activated when the cell needs to replicate to continue keeping the organism alive.

The many receptors on the surface of every cell control how that cell functions. Cell receptors send signals to the bloodstream, letting the body know what the cell needs. The cell receptors also respond to the influences of our environment, toxins, nutrition and even our thoughts and emotions.

How do the cells know what's going on in the rest of the body and beyond? The key is the interstitial fluid that surrounds every cell and, via the molecules in this fluid, links each cell with the rest of the body and with the external environment. The nervous system 'reads' environmental signals which are interpreted by our brain and a host of nerve fibres in our skin, lungs and gastrointestinal tract. The brain releases chemicals (e.g. hormones, neurotransmitters, growth factors), which are carried in the blood, along with the metabolised elements from our food and the air we breathe. The blood travels through increasingly smaller vessels, until it reaches the fluid around every cell, the 'interstitial sea'. The cell receptors then mediate an exchange of nutrients and waste products depending on the needs of every individual cell in the body. Clever, eh?

Cell receptors make the best decisions they can for the survival of the organism, moment by moment, adapting to what is happening in the interstitial sea, which is actually a connection to the whole body.

---

[2] Bruce Lipton (2005) *Biology of Belief*. Hay House: US

> In 2005, our second granddaughter, Claire, was born in Seattle, US and, while we stayed with my daughter and her family, I listened to a radio broadcast by Dr Bruce Lipton. Bruce was speaking on the local radio about his new book called *The Biology of Belief.* I was incredibly excited to hear out loud what I had been thinking about because his science made so much sense to me! My daughter told me that we could ring the radio station and speak with him. I opened the conversation with, 'Dr Lipton, you wrote my book!' An hour later, I hung up, feeling a sense of hope and the promise of a bright future. Dr Lipton continues his work today and I highly recommend that you check out his website.[3]

## Molecules of emotion

What we eat, drink, breathe or absorb in any other way changes our interstitial fluid and can affect our health. Moment by moment, we secrete a sea of chemistry in accordance with our thinking and feeling. The secreted molecules of emotion are the 'issues in our tissues'.

This concept, that Candace Pert first explored and translated into readable science,[4] challenged the conventional theory that stress is all in the mind and does not affect how the body works. You only have to remember the last time you felt 'butterflies in the stomach' to realise that this makes no sense!

Short-term stress can be good for us, to motivate us to do something that needs to be done. The body goes into 'fight or flight' mode, releasing messenger molecules (*neurotransmitters*) such as cortisol, that

---

[3] https://www.brucelipton.com
[4] Candace B Pert (1997). *Molecules of Emotion: The Science Behind Mind Body Medicine.* Simon and Schuster: US.

tell the cells to make extra energy and prepare for action. However, feeling stressed for a long period of time and having chronically high levels of stress hormones disrupts the body's processes and negatively affects our health.

What has this got to do with cancer? If the body is challenged by unrelenting stress, physical deprivation or emotional abuse and our cells are bombarded with the chemistry of our 'fight or flight' mode, the immune system becomes suppressed and cancer cells can take hold. I see it as a kind of 'chemical inflammation' caused by stress that generally happens over a long time.

Of course, there are many positive messenger molecules too! A great piece of research came out about eight years ago and many reputable studies have followed,[5] showing that positive chemicals (e.g. endorphins) that we secrete during and after exercise are the same as those that are produced in response to pleasurable pursuits such as laughing, singing and massage. These 'happy' chemicals create a well-nurtured immune system that can help to restore us to health if disease is present.

Of course, I am not suggesting that 'happiness' can cure cancer. There are many medically advisable treatment options that give us the best shot of overcoming cancer. Modern cancer treatments like chemotherapy, radiation and surgery 'de-bulk' the number of cancer cells in the body and often eliminate them altogether. If we confidently make peace with our chosen treatment, we lower our 'stress chemistry'. If somewhere along the cancer treatment road we find moments of gratitude and perhaps bliss, we can even boost our immune system.

Every cell in the body is seeking balance and health (*homeostasis*). Our immune system is designed to identify which cells are allowed to prosper and replicate and which cells are eliminated because they are

---

[5] https://www.physio.co.uk/treatments/massage/physiological-effects-of-massage/hormonal-effects/increased-endorphines-serotonin-dopamine.php/

https://www.health.harvard.edu/staying-healthy/exercising-to-relax

abnormal. When our immune system falls asleep, the abnormal cells go unchecked, they prosper and we can become sick. This happens from conception to death. Our immune system is the key to health and longevity.

*Anandamide* is the ultimate 'happy' molecule of emotion. In Sanskrit, *ananda* means bliss. Anandamide is the hormone we make naturally when we feel a 'sense of bliss', whether by making love, holding a baby as it sleeps, listening to the roar of a Formula One engine… whatever is uniquely blissful for us. Massage and meditation are wonderful bliss promoters! Anandamide *potentiates* the cell, making it the best cell it can be. Interestingly, the active ingredient in cannabis attaches to the anandamide receptor, blocking the receptor site to our 'homemade' anandamide. When people use cannabis, it latches onto the receptor and provides an altered state of relaxation, even though there is no benefit to the wellbeing of the cell.

## The relaxation response

Relaxation and bliss are essential for a healthy body. Relaxation is interesting biology which I first encountered in the early 1970s. When I was growing up, people were sent to convalescent hospitals to recover after medical treatment, especially surgery. The aim of convalescence was to breathe fresh air, eat wholesome food and sleep a lot – 'bliss' for a body recovering from early anaesthetic chemicals like ether, surgical wounds and workplaces that expected a fully functional worker on their return to work following treatment.

Things are certainly different now, and most of us expect to function at a high level no matter what is going on in our bodies. Over time, this can take a toll on our physical and mental health. True relaxation is essential to our wellbeing and there is a process in our nervous system that passes on the benefits to the whole body. It is our relaxation response. It is the opposite of the 'fight or flight' response and, through the release of positive neurotransmitters such as serotonin and dopamine, it gives our cells the message that we are safe and all is well.

Dr Herbert Benson published a little red book in 1975 describing the biology of the relaxation response.[6] He described how meditation alone, undertaken by experienced practitioners, brought about 'striking physiological changes – decreased heart rate, metabolic rate, and breathing rate'. It has since been shown that relaxation dilates blood vessels enough to lower blood pressure. Meditation, breathing exercises, progressive muscle relaxation, yoga and massage have all been shown to induce this relaxation response.

## Mind-body connection

Candace Pert's work also showed that the body and mind are one. If our cells are affected, not just by what we put into or onto our bodies, but also by our thoughts and emotions, then the mind and body must be intimately connected and constantly communicating with each other. This challenged the traditional Western belief that it is only the brain that secretes neurotransmitters. It is clear that these messenger molecules arise in both the body and the brain and messages are transmitted in both directions, influencing cell function when they latch onto cell receptor sites.

At JCSMR in the mid-1980s, I was involved in isolating nerve growth factors found in beef heart, and I took a keen interest in Pert's work. It was different from everything I had learned up until that point, and it was certainly very exciting. It also made sense of my personal experience (research data of ONE).

---

[6] Herbert Benson (1975) The Relaxation Response. HarperTorch (reissue edition, 2000).

Ten days before I was married, I had my appendix taken out at St Vincent's Hospital in Sydney. I had just resigned from my job there and after our honeymoon in Noosa, we travelled to Jervis Bay Naval College where Chris had been posted. After 18 months, I returned to the histology department at St Vincent's and immediately looked up my appendix slides in the filing cabinet – NAD (no abnormalities detected). So, what had caused 'that' pain, a pain severe enough for the surgeon to remove my appendix?

I felt the same pain in my side again when I was living briefly with my parents 13 years later. We were just about to leave for PNG, Chris was at a language course in Melbourne and our daughters were attending my old primary school. It was too long after my appendix operation to feel adhesions for the first time, so I ignored 'that' pain and carried on.

Six years later, I was running a meditation group at my local church – a passion for me and a challenge for the minister we had at the time. Each week, I persevered with a small group of folk seeking peace of mind. After a forceful talk from the minister, as I sat in silent meditation, 'that' pain returned.

In the peace of meditation, I realised that each time I was in a super stressful situation, the area of my body where my appendix once lived, hurt like crazy. This was mind-body medicine coming alive in my own experience.

Over the ensuing decades, science expanded and enriched my understanding of my physical experiences and those of my massage clients. Fast forward to now, the body-mind connection has finally become accepted by the medical community!

This 'heart transplant' story is very interesting. Research undertaken by the Heart Math Institute (www.heartmath.com) over 25 years shows that more messages travel from the heart to the brain than the other way around, influencing brain functions like clarity of mind and emotions. When a 12-year-old girl was given the heart of a murdered 12-year-old girl, the recipient of the heart could give enough evidence to convict the killer of her donor. The heart rules the body. Recently I listened to a Radio National book review of *Can You Die of a Broken Heart?* – you sure can!

Candace Pert wrote, 'I seek to inform, to educate, to inspire all manner of people, from lay to professional,' and she did. However, after she died in 2013, her voice grew 'soft' in the science community, though her work lives on. I hope that another loud voice emerges soon. I believe that mind-body chemistry is the foundation and cornerstone of healing.

Chapter 12 provides practical information about what we can all do to help our immune systems, minds and bodies.

### Bringing science and massage together

So, how does OM fit in with this science?

> I clearly remember a couple from out west in NSW. He had an upper left lobe lung lesion and his upper chest was warm to my touch. His wife asked me if she could watch the treatment so she could help him when they got home. Of course, I agreed. I did mainly fascial release and then very gentle OM on his whole body. As I finished the treatment, his wife asked if she could feel the 'warm patch'. We both did and it had disappeared entirely. His whole chest felt the same temperature, he was no longer in pain and his face was relaxed and almost wrinkle-free.

I took my observations to respected colleagues with many years of experience in science and tactile therapies. The consensus was that my treatment had unblocked a 'traffic jam' of immune helper cells and the like, allowing the interstitial sea to decongest. The relaxation in his facial features was just that, the relaxation response we talked about before, and the work of the bliss hormone, anandamide, potentiating the cells.

## What is the published evidence?

In 2004, Cassileth and Vickers (Memorial Sloan Kettering Cancer Centre [MSKCC] New York) published results of a large study on 'light touch' massage that has stood the test of time:[7]

- Pain improved by 47 per cent;
- Fatigue improved by 42 per cent;
- Anxiety improved by 59 per cent;
- Nausea improved by 51 per cent;
- Depression improved by 48 per cent; and
- Other side effects like shortness of breath, memory problems, dry mouth or disturbed sleep improved by 48 per cent.

Peer-reviewed, published studies from reputable institutions around the world have confirmed the 2004 MSKCC study, although most are too small to be considered 'high quality' in medical terms.

There are small observational studies like the one by Gai Walker, a palliative care nurse and OM therapist from East Gippsland, Victoria, who conducted her own research measuring oxygen saturation, pulse, blood pressure and respiration pre- and post-OM. Massage of this type consistently demonstrated a positive shift in physiological measures and a clinical benefit to clients. Gai's data is available on request.

---

[7] Barrie R Cassileth, Andrew J Vickers (2004) *Massage therapy for symptom control: outcome study at a major cancer centre.* J Pain Symptom Manage; 28(3): 244-9.

Frustrated with the lack of Australian data, in 2016, I approached Western Sydney University (WSU) to partner with OML to undertake a study into the current use of complementary therapies, such as massage in cancer services.

OM therapists around Australia, trained by OMT and OML, were instrumental in encouraging hospitals to complete the WSU survey as they had developed strong relationships with them based on positive patient outcomes, and there was an amazing 92 per cent participation rate by cancer services throughout Australia.

In 2018, WSU published a paper showing that 72 per cent of cancer patients wanted massage as their preferred complementary medicine (CM) therapy.[8] The paper showed that OM can change the way people feel about living with a serious illness. By providing clinically reasoned and thoughtfully adapted massage, therapists nourish body, mind and spirit to:

- Improve quality of life
- Reduce anxiety
- Help with pain management
- Improve quality of sleep
- Reduce fatigue
- Reduce unpleasant sensations from chemotherapy-induced peripheral neuropathy (CIPN)
- Increase function in areas affected by scar tissue resulting from surgery and radiation
- Reduce post-surgical swelling and support rehabilitation and recovery
- Support the lymph system and assist with lymphedema management
- Improve body image awareness

---

[8] J Hunter, J Ussher, C Parton, A Kellett, C Smith, G Delaney, E Oyston (2018) *Australian Integrative Oncology Services: a mixed-method study exploring the views of cancer survivors.* BMC Complementary and Alternative Medicine; 18(10): 153.

Follow-up research may be happening around the country regarding OM, however I have not had any enquiries to date.

**And now… a rant!**

If I were to repeat my time in science, I would like to work with the mind-body aspect of immunomodulatory treatments – to find ways of boosting the production of natural killer (NK) lymphocytes and test for neurotransmitters, peptides, ligands and hormones produced by love, laughter and gentle massage… OM!

Unfortunately, it seems that 'new' ideas like OM, meditation and acupuncture, even when established by sound medical research and carried out in highly regarded institutions, are often met with scepticism and obstructive discourse.

How medicine understands cells, nutrients and biological pathways changes constantly. The medical model of drug therapy, radiotherapy and surgery is the best educated guess of medical science and is increasingly successful because of continuing scientific advances. Complementary medicine is also based on current scientific understanding, viewed from a different angle.

There is not one way to cure cancer – if there was, we would all share the good news. There is, however, the hope that we can view new ideas with vision and curiosity. We need all the science and miracles of medicine *and* complementary medicine.

What if massage was offered to help patients having an adverse chemotherapy reaction, as I saw recently on an ABC documentary about the Chris O'Brien Lifehouse in Sydney? The OM calmed the patient, lowered their blood pressure and brought their heart back into a gentle rhythm. This small segment of the documentary filled me with hope.

Massage is a powerful experience for a person who believes that they are too sick to be touched. OM offers safe, gentle touch to everyone without judgement. Even when folk are very ill, there is a place where a hand can touch with compassion and kindness. This is not 'new-age' thinking; it is excellent medical science.

# 3.

# The Power of Compassionate Touch

All of this new science brought together what had been dawning on me over two decades of looking down a microscope. At the same time that I was marvelling at the neuroscience and absorbing the implications for how I now understood the body, I went to massage school to learn the practicalities of putting my hands onto mostly healthy people. Then I began massaging participants on the QFL cancer programs and it was there that I found a language to express my intuition.

This was a time of huge self-discovery and deep emotional change. I developed a new awareness of myself, an understanding of others and how life experience influences choices about cancer management and treatment. Finally, I developed massage skills based on scientific understanding and absorbed an ocean of new information from both the medical and complementary therapy communities.

What I learned from observing cancer in the laboratory and then as a part of life for many people (including me), is that I am not afraid of cancer, I'm curious. Not 'why me?' but 'why not me?' and if it is me, why now? What is it in my experience of life that has put my immune system to sleep, long enough for these cells to grow and flourish undetected and stop me in my tracks? Or does the sea of chemical challenges we all face eventually overwhelm our safekeeping mechanisms?

The momentum for my journey of learning and amalgamating new and old information was the growing need for safe, gentle, compassionate touch in our society, especially when we are vulnerable and frightened.

### The seeds had already been sown

Despite being spent in impersonal labs, my years as a scientist taught me about the implications of test results on peoples' lives. I had learned a great deal more than what we saw down the microscope. I had prepared patients for procedures like bone marrow biopsy, witnessing their fear and apprehension, and managed specimens through the laboratory process. I then sat with the pathologist while the most probable diagnosis was determined. All of my training in haematology, histology and cytology happened this way so it was a comprehensive apprenticeship.

> One Christmas Eve, I was the technician on duty. I ran all the liquid laboratory tests knowing that the blood film was urgent, so I called in the haematologist and we sat together to look at a cell population that represented acute myeloid leukaemia. The patient was 12 years old. In that moment, I realised that I was the first to see 'life-changing cells' and that what I wrote on my report, to be countersigned by the pathologist, would change the lives of a whole family, a school and a neighbourhood forever. I was 19 years old.

For much of this time, I floated along feeling confused as I didn't have the language to express myself and the laboratory culture didn't encourage us to 'feel'. We were stoic and professional. It took me another 20 years to find teachers in my western culture who wrote about the philosophy of health and cultural attitudes to healing.

## Massage school – something completely different

Even with my emerging awareness, massage school took me by surprise. It was an 'oo-me-goo-me-la-la' experience for a scientist – cabbages planted by the cycles of the moon, diseases linked to emotions, acupuncture meridians and foot reflexology. Foot reflexology? What the heck is that about? I sat at the back of the class wondering why I was even there.

Upholding scientific integrity while embarking on a journey of discovery – what to keep and what to discard – felt tricky at first. Maintaining curiosity in the face of something that doesn't fit with what you have always believed brings interest alive and makes it real.

When I look back over my 'road less travelled', I notice that, somehow, I was in the right place at the right time, learning the lessons that prepared me for what was to come.

Massage school was where I first noticed how 'bliss' changes our physiology. In the student clinic, where clients pay a nominal fee and the students do a supervised massage, I noticed the marked difference in people's facial expressions before and after the session.

In my student clinic experience, clients received remedial massages for musculoskeletal problems. I was taught not to massage people with a systemic disease like diabetes or cancer, heart disease or neurodegenerative diseases (like Parkinson's disease). This is of course impossible to do – systemic diseases are unavoidable if we massage a cross-section of the public, including those aged over 65 years. Every health professional is taught how to do a thorough intake questionnaire, however not every client will answer truthfully.

## Discovering fascia

While I was at massage school, I heard about Bowen therapy (BT), an Australian bodywork technique developed by the late Tom Bowen (1916-1982). Tom lived in Geelong, Victoria, and was widely known across Australia. Legend has it that he didn't make appointments so there was a queue of cars in his street from early morning until late at night.

Tom's memory continues to be honoured by therapists in Australia and around the world. If you have ever used his techniques, you will know he was a genius, years ahead of his time.

I studied a brand of BT called fascial kinetics, developed by Russell Sturgess. Russell was originally a massage therapist who studied Chinese medicine before exploring and making scientific sense of BT. Russell taught the science of fascia long before fascial research burst into medical awareness (around 2007). There is a wealth of information available now about fascia and the importance of hydration to a healthy body.

I loved the science of fascia, which was new to me. The way Russell taught the work of Candace Pert (Molecules of Emotion) and the outcomes I saw in others sparked my curiosity. BT courses are very practical. Students pair up and practise techniques on one another. At first, I didn't feel the changes in my own body that I witnessed in the other students, and I was forced to conclude that maybe I was so full of toxins that I couldn't feel any of the very subtle changes that this very gentle technique facilitates.

Now, I can definitely feel my body change when I undergo a BT treatment. Many of the Bowen moves are over acupuncture points, where the fascia tracks downwards to the periosteum (the tough, thin outer membrane covering all the bones of the body). Muscles, ligaments and tendons attach to the periosteum. The periosteum has a close connection to the immune system.

BT combines brilliantly with OM and offers a future of safe, respectful touch, based on compassion.

### Fascia and hydration

A relatively recent addition to routine health advice is to drink 1.5 to 2 litres of water each day. When I was growing up, drinking sugar-laden fizzy drinks was actively encouraged!

Staying hydrated is all about lubricating our fascia.

Inside our bodies, fascia fills all the spaces between the skin and the muscles, and the muscles and the organs. Fascia called 'mesentery' links the loops of our intestines in a particular way so they don't get tangled.

Fascia is called the 'web of life' and when it is hydrated, nutrients move effortlessly around the body and we feel healthy. When we become dehydrated for any reason (even sitting in a hot car in summer), the distribution of nutrients is inhibited and, more importantly, so is the elimination of metabolism by-products like urea. We feel terrible.

Fascia was poorly understood until scanning electron microscopy, mid last century, revealed the mystery of how fluid and immune system cells travel around the body via the fascia.

I learned about fascia through touch. Fascia is palpable and thermal (the skin temperature changes in different parts of the body) and therapists can feel when it is dehydrated or 'glued'. In OM we teach a 'global shoulder release' that is based on releasing shoulder fascia.

After radiotherapy or surgery for any upper body tumour, the large and complex shoulder fascia can become 'sticky' and tight (commonly called 'frozen shoulder'), making the global shoulder release technique gently therapeutic. Scar release techniques taught in OM are also based on gentle fascial release.

> I was invited to demonstrate OM scar techniques to the teachers at a Southern Sydney massage school where we were running OM courses. The client they chose for my demonstration had had regular massage since her radical mastectomy 18 months before. A skilled, experienced, remedial massage (RM) therapist had regularly worked on releasing her shoulder fascia and the tightness in her neck, however the gains were short-lived. The woman's scars were neat but extensive. Her left axilla (armpit) was holding fluid and by the end of the day, she was often in pain and had trouble sleeping.
>
> They had given me their 'too hard basket' challenge for a one-hour demonstration!
>
> I began with gentle OM of her hips and lower back, I did some light stroking of the axilla, both arms, a global shoulder release on both sides, and then gently worked the scar fascia. An hour later, the client was waving her arms around claiming that I'd cured her! A week later her RM therapist rang me to say that the improvements I'd achieved (much the same as she had over the past 18 months) were holding. A month later she rang again, and they were still holding. What had I done? I can't explain it scientifically, but I can show you!

I could write a whole book about fascia! If you're interested in knowing more, look for the textbook *Job's Body* by Deane Juhan,[9] as well as the work of Dr Robert Schleip in Germany.[10]

---

[9] Deane Juhan (1987) *Job's body: a Handbook for Bodywork*. Station Hill Press: New York.
[10] Podcast interview with Dr Robert Schleip https://www.youtube.com/watch?v=PVoNR_coiyM

## Arriving at Quest for Life – the scales fell off

My time at QFL was so intense and full of memories, it is hard to recall with any clarity. It was a rollercoaster of a time for me. I was full of new knowledge, practised in doing remedial massage on mostly healthy people and passionate about fascia. It was at QFL that everything came together for me.

Within a short time, I realised that touch for people living with illness of any kind must be gentle. Even when folk came to me in the massage room with sciatica or a frozen shoulder, as well as cancer, they were yearning for safe, gentle human touch.

All the participants at QFL had their own cancer story, with their partners or a loved one caring for them. The groups were small by today's standards and the team was generous – two facilitators, two support people, two massage therapists and a gifted counsellor who took emotional care of us all.

When the co-facilitator moved away, I asked Petrea if she would give me a go at co-facilitating with her.

Poignant memories are often confused with myths and wishes so the following story is my 'best guess'.

> As the co-facilitator of the cancer program part of my responsibility was to care for the participants overnight, so when my phone rang at 2 am the support person and I made our way to the guest's bedroom.
>
> A woman in her early 50s with advanced cancer had severe abdominal pain. She had taken all the drugs her doctors had prescribed and put heat packs around her back and abdomen. She and her partner, with a lifetime of experience, both looked like 'deer in the headlights' and said, 'Please don't make us go to hospital. We just want this last weekend together.'

> I don't really know why – to give myself time to assess the situation, I imagine – I knelt beside the bed, slipped my hands under the doona and rested them on her rock-hard abdomen. Then I waited and the tension in the room slowly lessened. I don't recall how long I gently held my hands on her tummy. Eventually her abdomen began to soften and we all felt much more relaxed.
>
> I applied lotion to her abdomen gently for about 20 minutes and she drifted into sleep. I tucked the couple into bed and put out the light.
>
> The next morning, we walked to the chemist together and she asked me what I did to stop the pain. I don't know exactly, as there was no double-blind research project to advise me. Instead, I followed my instincts and brought 'human potential' and compassion to the moment.

This is one of the many stories that guided me to write an OM training program. Once I knew, deep inside my soul, the power of skilled gentle massage I wanted everyone to experience the benefits of deep relaxation and safe touch.

## Sharing the science

I had a good reason for wanting to explain the science of cancer to participants on our programs. Again, my observational research of one! In 1985, Chris' dad was in an aged care facility and very close to the end of his life. He had prostate cancer.

> Grandfather was not my favourite person as he had never approved of our marriage. My parents were not rich enough for his youngest son and we came from the wrong part of town – migrant heaven, the western suburbs of Sydney. We hadn't seen much of Les over the years as he was well cared for by Chris' oldest brother, but he came to us for two enjoyable and memorable holidays.
>
> In the nursing home, he was old, sad and very fragile. Chris left to pick up some toiletries and snacks and Les looked me in the eye. 'You wear a white coat?' 'Yes, I do.' 'Did I get prostate cancer because I was promiscuous in my youth?' 'No, Les, you didn't.' 'How did the cancer get to my bones?' I picked up his cigarette packet and drew a sketch of how metastatic spread was thought to occur in 1985.
>
> When Chris came back his first remark was, 'What did you say to Dad? He looks so peaceful.'

Not everyone wants to know how cancer grows and spreads, but everyone wants reassurance. Gentle, honest compassion can be expressed verbally as well as physically.

When I was diagnosing cancer as a cytotechnologist, many a dinner party conversation centred on my job. I knew that some people needed to know about their diagnosis or illness in a very specific way. Remember how I needed to look at my appendix slides when I had the chance months after my surgery? My brand of curiosity is a need to see and understand.

I enjoyed sharing simplified science and answering whatever questions I could for friends and family. I always made it very clear that my comments were based on my experience and, if my words worried them in any way, they must check it out with their medical team.

As I shared my 'brand' of science with more and more participants at QFL, the more exciting it became. Petrea is a first-class researcher, and she generously shared her findings with me. I did my very best to help answer questions that a medical team was too busy to answer, or the person felt were too silly or trivial to ask. These are the questions that keep people awake at night, feed the worry and fear cycle and steal their peace. We can never go back to the day before we are told we have cancer.

## At the beginning – a dream

> My dream was that every oncologist had a lovely room next to their consulting room, where I could take people after their medical consultation, particularly the first one.
>
> I imagined a safe, peaceful place for people to explore their feelings after what they had just heard – a diagnosis of cancer. People could cry, scream, feel relief (as some would finally know what was wrong with them), or sit in stunned silence and shock... 'Me? I have cancer?' And ask all the 'silly' questions they needed to ask, for as long as it took. This would be patient-centred care at its best!

Sadly, the concept of 'patient-centred care' wasn't talked about at cancer conferences for another 15 years. Even now, 'support' nurses are present but so time-poor that patients are often left feeling confused and alone. They often resort to getting answers from the internet or from ill-informed friends.

Before patients left my imaginary room, they would have a gentle, mindful massage to centre them and help them to begin reconnecting with themselves. The massage could start the process of seeking a 'new normal', a new relationship with their body... a body in need of healing and peace.

If only kindness and compassionate touch were affordable. To create my little 'support' room, I needed space and time. Medical office space is unaffordable, and I would need to 'volunteer' my time. How would I eat, provide for my family or pay professional costs like insurance?

There had to be another way.

In 2001, at a meeting of the Australian Traditional Medicine Society (ATMS), I was excited by an aromatherapist's lecture telling us that massage and pure essential oils were safe to use on clients with cancer and heart disease. The speaker based her talk on research by Tiffany Field in the US.[11] This was what I needed; the beginnings of evidence-based research to underpin my deep knowing.

However, there were so many questions whirling around my mind! What if the recently discovered chemical therapies, now common for treating cancer, interacted with the aromatherapy essences? What would the medical and pharmaceutical community make of that idea? How could I develop oncology massage training that integrated respectfully with the current medical model? Would massage offered to people with cancer from diagnosis to the end of life ever be supported by their medical team?

Was I still dreaming? I knew the power of safe, gentle touch, and that passion and compassion can change everything.

## Developing Massage, Cancer and More

Speaking with experienced massage therapists at QFL, yoga and meditation teachers and Wendie Batho (Petrea's partner), I started to write an OM training program. When I asked around for ideas for the title of my course Petrea suggested 'Massage, Cancer and More' (MC&M).

---

[11] Touch Research Institute, University of Miami/Miller School of Medicine, US; Fielding Graduate University, US.

I actually cannot remember much about the early course content. It is almost 20 years since I did this work and all the adjustments, fine-tuning, accreditation and medical ethics committee changes happened over time. When I wrote the first manual, I was mostly alone.

I wrote articles for every massage journal and natural therapies newsletter willing to print my story, promoting OM as the conduit or pathway for complementary modalities into mainstream medical services.

I continue to hold this belief. In 2022, OM research is available. Every new study affirms what MSKCC wrote about in 2004. OM is safe, effective, well-researched and cost-effective. To this day, I need money to make the practice happen more widely in our embattled medical system.

## Learning from Gayle MacDonald

Gayle MacDonald was a founder of oncology massage in the US. Three years after I started teaching MC&M (2008), Gayle came to QFL to support me and teach the finer points of oncology massage training. She shared her experience of integrated complementary medicine and supported or guided my ideas.

Gayle loves to teach beginners and her program is a fantastic experience. Gayle's spirituality and medical knowledge guides her every word – an OM technique intensive that validated and enriched my work. I am very fortunate that my program evolved under her expert eye.

I did Gayle's foundation course twice at QFL as her assistant. A year later, I travelled to Portland, Oregon, to undertake Gayle's in-hospital program before I wrote and developed in-hospital training in Australia (OM3 and OM4, see Chapter 7).

Gayle remains the dearest of friends, and her role in OM in the US, Australia and Europe, especially Scotland, is a significant part of

## The Power of Compassionate Touch

her life's work. Together we dreamed about holding international conferences in The Netherlands, the 'centre' of the OM world as we knew it.

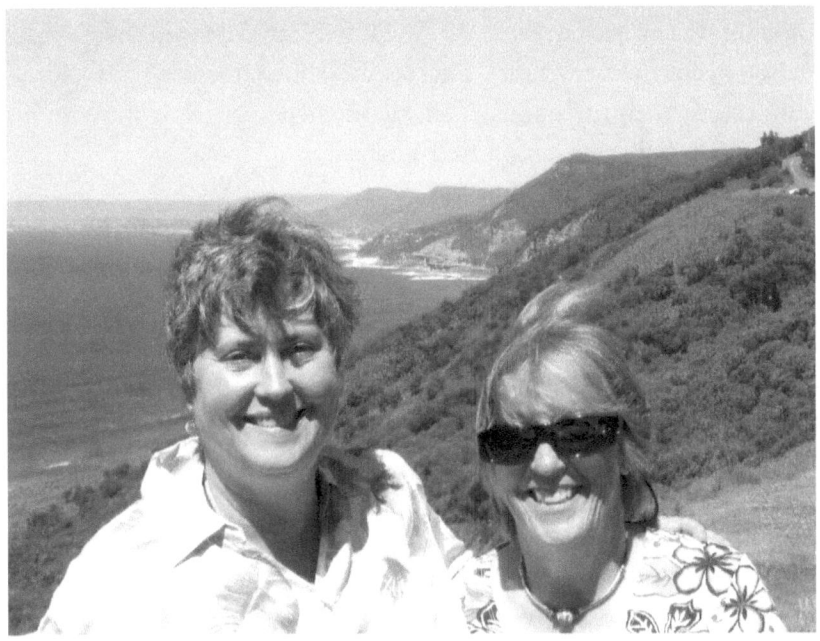

Gayle's first day in Australia.

### First things first

The best way to train massage therapists is to let them experience the event or feeling, and with any luck, they will modify what they were taught in massage school to incorporate the new, gentler methods of touching clients. An important part of this is being mindful and centred on the client.

By watching Petrea work, I learned how to put my thoughts and fears aside and be totally present. Most of the things that hold us in fear are thoughts of the future that haven't happened yet and may never happen, or memories of experiences from our past, often seen through the eyes of the child or teenager we still carry inside us.

Russell, my first Bowen teacher, taught me to imagine that every client lying on the massage table could see a TV screen, onto which my every thought was projected. Such as, 'What will I make for dinner?', 'This person needs to lose weight,' 'I'm so scared of her disease I'm avoiding connecting with my hands,' etc. He insisted that we work without judgement, busyness, fear or self-interest.

Gayle MacDonald's program includes a practical demonstration of this concept which I adapted for the first OM module (see Chapter 5).

## What did I need to teach?

MC&M was based on the science I taught in my pathophysiology course, the gentle massage techniques I used with my clients and how to look after myself when working with folk on the edge of life, balanced with what I learned about myself at QFL. It was a simple three-day course, 24 hours (plus a few hours crammed into late nights) of theory and practise. There is more about the course content in Chapter 5.

There were no rules and no instructions in 2002, just my golden rule – gentle, focused and non-judgmental. Even when you are faced with many contraindications, there is *always* somewhere you can touch with compassion. Hold a head gently, caress a foot.

## The early days

The first MC&M course was at QFL. It was a large group of about 12 therapists, including five memorable folk from Eastern Palliative Care in Melbourne and a senior nurse from a major hospital in Sydney. It was a week-long residential program and all the beautiful resources at QFL were made available.

The Melbourne therapists were experienced and generously added to the practical sessions with advice, stories and tips on home-based OM compared with massage clinic OM sessions.

I quickly learned how important a community of like-minded people is when you are flying at the outer edge of medical and massage industry norms.

> The senior nurse was interesting. I had carefully vetted qualifications and insurance documents for all the students; to be included they needed two years' experience massaging healthy clients with musculoskeletal issues. She met the criteria. I said to the group, 'Set up tables and whoever is on the table needs to go down to their underwear.' She whispered in my ear, with surprise, that she was not going to do that!
>
> All her massage training had been done online and she had not attended a single practical session to achieve her qualification. I was feeling cross when I told her she couldn't continue the program unless she was prepared to give and receive the practical component of MC&M. She stayed and learned a great deal.

This course was the first time I assessed a Shiatsu therapist. The only way I could think to do that was for her to imagine I had right breast cancer with lymph nodes fully excised, treat me accordingly and see what I felt. All I really knew about Shiatsu was that it was based on traditional Chinese medicine (TCM) principles. I had some understanding of acupuncture and meridians as I had done a 12-day Tuina TCM course in China in 2001. The Shiatsu therapist treated me to a wonderful experience of relaxation and deep fascial release. She became an OM teacher and therapist of an exceptional standard (she was one of the two therapists employed by the Chris O'Brien Lifehouse, Sydney, when it opened) and I count her as a dear friend to this day.

After paying QFL the venue costs, I still had money left for advertising and I selected dates and cities where therapists had shown interest. I took speaking engagements at Darling Harbour Natural Therapies Expo, Sutherland Library, ATMS Conference, Natural Therapy Expo in Brisbane, in fact I spoke to anybody who would listen! Before long I was teaching in Melbourne with students from as far away as Central Queensland and New Zealand, Sydney and Surfer's Paradise, Queensland.

Even from this humble beginning, I knew I had something of value. Many folk have wanted to take my work and use it for financial gain but none have done it. Some have incorporated my work into massage school courses without acknowledgement or permission, and with no advanced science or any experience of massaging people with cancer or a history of cancer. There isn't a regulator to make training organisations accountable, unless they are prepared to register with S4OM in the US. In the beginning, I hoped that massage associations and insurance companies would control who was eligible to work in a hospital or medical practice to ensure that they were properly trained, but this didn't happen either.

I have never been able to rein in the arrogant folk who think that gentle massage is simple, 'do no harm' stuff.

## Learning on the go

The merry-go-round of teaching MC&M was exhausting.

> It was my first course in Brisbane and a trusted friend suggested I use an affordable hotel on the edge of the city. Only three therapists enrolled, and I booked the penthouse to accommodate us as well as providing a teaching space. I shared my room with a student to save money. I walked to the nearest shops to

> buy food and water and lugged it all up the hill as I couldn't stop a taxi.
>
> The therapists were curious, and I noticed the 'vacuum cleaner' on my brain for the first time.
>
> I included meals in the deal (like QFL, my gold standard) and either cooked organic food or took them out for a meal in the city. They all raved about the course – value for money and a great learning experience. They were stoked, and at 55 years old, I took a week to recover. It would kill me now at 73!

The goal of this exercise was to show the OM therapists that they were valued professionals. In the early 2000s, the massage therapy profession, in the minds of the public, was tainted by association with the sex industry. This has been a very hard perception to shift, and even today, young therapists are occasionally asked for a 'happy ending'.

Smarter than before the Brisbane fiasco, the next course I remember clearly was in Canberra. This time I rented two apartments, one for teaching and one for sleeping and eating. I recruited Chris to make the meals and also look after a carer who needed a rest. She was a health professional who got great benefit from sharing meals with the massage students and talking about her physical and emotional experience as a carer for her young husband with advanced bowel cancer. This was a great lesson for the OM therapists-in-training.

While running courses and working at QFL, I also set up an 'issues in your tissues' clinic in Canberra with Trish, my dear friend and colleague. We worked together until my OM travel took me away too often and I left the practice. Trish is from 'out west', a career nurse who became a massage and BT therapist. She is the best therapist I have ever worked with and her commitment to her clients brings them back to her clinic for years.

I never set out to 'build a business'; I set out to respectfully let the medical world know that massage, the right kind of massage, could bring comfort and relaxation to very sick people. I was on a steep learning curve with high ideals and dreams of doing whatever it took to get the job done. My problem was I didn't identify the 'job', I just rolled along from one course to the next, learning along the way and running myself into the ground.

They say you teach what you need to learn!

## MC&M becomes OMT

In my work running programs for people with cancer and their partners, I noticed the needs of carers. Carers or family members often wanted to touch, massage or cuddle the person with cancer but were too scared of doing harm, so they didn't. I decided to include people without massage training in a modified MC&M that became OM1. The first time I did this was in a Brisbane course, with an architect married to a naturopath with advanced mouth cancer. He picked up massage skills easily, as well as what 'gentle' could achieve, even though he was learning massage and OM skills from scratch. This was a timely lesson for me. Bowen therapists were enrolling in my programs and appeared to be perfect OM students even though they did not have Swedish or remedial massage training. Later I learned about a fantastic program called 'Safe Touch for Carers' by William Collinge (US), filmed at MSKCC in New York with assistance from Tracy Walton, a co-founder of OM in the US. A video on YouTube offers a taste of this program.[12]

---

[12] William Collinge. Touch, Caring and Cancer: Simple Instruction for Family and Friends https://www.youtube.com/watch?v=n76wi9v74Pg

By now, I had realised that I needed help during the practical sessions in the programs. Two amazing therapists bubbled up from the 50 or so I had trained during MC&M and I began talking to them about teaching. They needed to have the training qualification I had achieved, Train the Trainer, before they started teaching OM and when they took that request on, I knew they would go the distance.

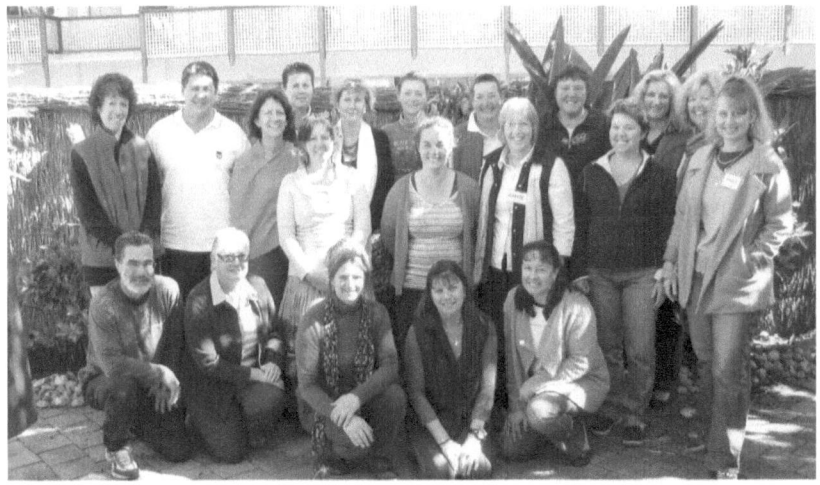

MC&M course Ballina, NSW, after Gayle's visit.
Tania Shaw, last on right, was my assistant

At every stage of developing the training modules, I learnt more about educational standards and how the rules worked. I implemented every 'rule', made them requirements for myself and others who wanted to teach OM as I needed this program to be a respected *bona fide* educational tool.

MC&M gradually became Oncology Massage Training (OMT), involving two three-day courses (Chapter 5). OM1 was open to anyone who wanted to learn gentle skills to help family or loved ones and as a foundation course for qualified massage therapists. OM2 was for massage professionals who wanted to advertise their new skills to local doctors and hospitals. OM3 and OM4 came later, for therapists who wanted to work in a medical setting (Chapters 6 and 7). Eventually, in 2013, OMT became OML, a registered charity.

OML continues to teach oncology massage courses now. It has been upgraded to meet current teaching requirements and MC&M remains the essence of the work. MC&M is also the basis of the OMG courses taught in Barcelona, Spain, and Buenos Aires, Argentina (Chapter 9).

This was another very busy time in my life! When I wasn't away teaching in major cities around Australia, I was working at QFL or massaging clients in Canberra or at home on the farm in Burra.

I sat behind the wheel of a car for many hours, which gave me plenty of time to think.

# 4.

# Debunking Some Myths

There are prevailing beliefs that stop oncology massage (OM) from being considered safe and effective for cancer patients. In a subtle way, massage has a growing presence in our community and medical system. However, few oncologists recommend massage for symptom management or quality of life challenges, even if they have read the US research or heard patients' endorsements of OM. Similarly, the view that massage has to reach the deep tissues of the body to provide therapeutic benefits may discourage people from considering OM if they are diagnosed with cancer.

Adding the word 'cancer' (or oncology) to massage elicits strong emotions in most people, much of which is about fear. Some people think that touch therapy has no place in active medical treatment – a world that is focused on quantity rather than quality of life. Some view massage as too onerous for frail bodies. Some even perpetuate the false idea that massage can spread cancer. It doesn't!

This chapter addresses some of these persistent myths and misconceptions.

## Touching frail bodies

Some people think, 'Could I have massaged Mum as she died?', sensing a missed opportunity to connect at the end of life, while others react as if we are suggesting touching the untouchable.

In the programs at QFL, Petrea King tells wonderful stories of 'holding' a person in pain, cradling the being, breathing in unison and acknowledging their suffering in the most intimate way. Families of those she supported attest to the joy and deep sense of communion this created, even in the most difficult of times.

Over the past 20 years, I have often experienced the power of deeply connecting with another who is suffering or dying. I shared the 'hands on the tummy at 2 am' story in the previous chapter and I 'held' my own mother in her final hours.

> The nurses brought me a reclining chair as the night wore on and Mum set about dying the way she wanted. During her 86th year of life, we had often talked about 'the end' and true to her feisty nature, she insisted 'I just want to slip away like my Dai' (Scots for father). That was exactly what came to pass and I saw it coming. At about 3 am, I decided to get into the hospital bed alongside Mum, hold her (the strongest memory from my childhood is being in her arms) and sing her an old Scottish tune, 'Oh but I'm longing for my aine folk'. The migrant journey never ends until it does. My mum 'slipped away' the following evening once I was safely surrounded by my own family. Her last words to me before she lapsed into unconsciousness were, 'I'll see you on the other side.'

Working with folk on the edge of life often directs conversation to death and dying, and I need you to know that massaging people with cancer has brought more laughter than tears. Real conversations that explore science, 'What will death be like?' or fractured relationships, 'How can I say sorry before I die?' and often the age-old question, 'Do you believe in God?' Often, tales of happier times fill the room with laughter and thanksgiving. What a privilege it has been to work as an OM therapist.

## Slow and steady versus 'no pain, no gain'

Although deep tissue massage in someone with a tumour does not spread cancer to other parts of the body, it is still unsafe for anyone with a life-changing disease. I think that strong remedial massage can cause the body to distribute 'defence chemicals', neurotransmitters that help us to manage the pain of these techniques. This might feel good in a healthy body with an uncompromised immune system, but it puts too much stress on a body with an immune system made vulnerable by disease, treatment side effects or age.

Release of muscles and fascia can be achieved with slow and gentle techniques (like OM and Bowen therapy) that can achieve 'deepness' without pain. These therapies, along with practices such as meditation, yoga, Feldenkrais and craniosacral release, give the body a better chance of pain relief by relaxing the muscles and gently stretching the fascia.[13,14]

The idea of releasing a tight 'trigger point' (a bundle of very thin muscle fibres that have 'stuck' together for some reason) with slow and gentle massage techniques, giving the muscle permission to release and disperse the stored lactic acid, will be hotly debated by many physiotherapists and remedial massage therapists.

---

[13] Herbert Benson (1975) The Relaxation Response. HarperTorch (reissue edition, 2000).
[14] Podcast interview with Dr Robert Schleip https://www.youtube.com/watch?v=PV0NR_coiyM

I don't have the money to prove my point with a double-blind research study. I do have 20 years of massage experience, observing excellent deep tissue muscle release with minimal or no pain. My clients appear relaxed, and their symptoms are reduced. They keep coming to my clinic because what I do 'helps' and, if they continue gentle treatment, long-term suffering eases and sometimes disappears. Often the 'no pain, no gain' methods stop folk from coming back because it hurts too much, so they give up hope, often relying just on pain relief medication.

The 'no pain, no gain' myth is the root of self-inflicted suffering. Like 'soldier on', this feeds into our modern myth that we are machines, ageless and invincible. Most massage schools teach musculoskeletal massage techniques that work best for fit athletes or younger people. I believe that the same relief of pain from muscle injury can be achieved with a gentle and deep technique, even in the young and fit. By treating only the injured area of the body, we miss the point. *Anatomy Trains* by Thomas Myers shows scientifically how we are fascially connected from the toes to the top of the head.[15] As our population ages and diseases like cancer and neurodegenerative conditions increase, our massage training must change.

OM can be offered to a client in cancer treatment or with a history of cancer, if the therapist has OM training by an S4OM accredited teacher or training organisation. Light body work techniques and gentle foot reflexology can bring comfort and connection. Bodies become fragile and vulnerable when disease, treatment drugs and fear dictate biology.

> I was working in the chemotherapy infusion room in a big Sydney hospital and the patient was a man in his mid-40s. He

---

[15] Myers, T (2009) Anatomy Trains: Myofascial Meridians for Manual and Movement Therapists. Churchill Livingstone Elsevier.

had just been diagnosed with advanced bowel cancer and his wife looked fearful and confused. I decided to gently rub his feet then do a shoulder release sequence. The foot work involved gentle foot reflexology, which I had learned in my massage training course and modified to ensure that my touch caused little or no pain. I sometimes started with this simple technique so I could talk to the clients a little more and explore their fears and experience around massage.

A month or so later, I was teaching at the same venue and the man passed me in a corridor. At the end of our chat, I asked if he had taken up the free foot reflexology sessions offered by the cancer support service. To my horror, he recoiled. The one treatment he had tried after mine was so painful he never tried massage again.

Deep tissue massage techniques pose the biggest obstacle to integrating massage into medical services and this is why I developed MC&M in 2001.

## Massage does *not* spread cancer

Cancer spreads biologically not mechanically. We cannot 'push' cancer around! Cancer spreads in the body whatever we are doing – watching TV, cooking, gardening, making love or exercising. Movement of healthy (or not so healthy) cells around the body is constant and moderated by neurochemicals and the functional demands of the body. As outlined in Chapter 2, the vitality of our immune system determines whether the cancer cell lives and flourishes or dies before it can become established and replicate.

The cell receptors on the cell surface have attachment points like a 'lock and key'. If the right 'lock' is not present the cancer cell cannot 'key' in. The cancer cell cannot stay and grow so it continues to look for a 'lock' that fits. Research from MSKCC showed that, when a cancer cell is travelling, it may not find a suitable site to 'lock' in until it gets back to the original cancer site.[16] This explains why some cancers seem to grow quickly. The cancer isn't a fast-growing 'oak tree', it's a 'bed of weeds' formed by the returning cancer cells. I love this imagery as it isn't too difficult to pull out a weed, but chopping down an oak tree is quite another task!

Massage does not play a part in the biological cancer process; our immune system does. Rather than spreading cancer, massage is much more likely to support the immune system by increasing endorphins and other positive hormones and eliciting the relaxation response.

I have been told by medical professionals that a morphine patch can reduce pain and anxiety for a mere 20 cents, so why should we spend money on oncology massage? In the medical world, OM is not cost-effective or time saving. However, morphine does not produce 'feel-good' chemicals like human touch does, nor does it potentiate the wellbeing of every cell like anandamide does.

What price do we put on compassionate touch?

## Cancer and fear

When I was a kid, cancer wasn't mentioned except in whispered tones. Even 20 years ago when I started MC&M, 'cancer' was a word that everyone feared. The underlying belief system based on fear is one of the emotional obstacles to cancer diagnosis and treatment, and often develops from an early age.

---

[16] Norton L, Massague J (2006). Is cancer a disease of self-seeding? *Nature Medicine* 12: 875-8.

> I remember being about 10 years old when our much-loved neighbour took ill. I heard the word 'cancer' and felt the emotions change around me. This neighbour used to invite me in on my way to school to do my hair. I loved her hairdo and I loved her. And then she was gone, and my morning excursions ended. I was told that she had died suddenly from 'some sort' of cancer treatment.

Children hear and feel everything, and when they don't understand they feel fear that usually stays with them throughout life.

Fear of being diagnosed, dying or losing a loved one, painful memories from treatment and emotions like loss, abandonment and anxiety restrict what is considered possible or appropriate for people with cancer.

A diagnosis of cancer, any cancer, changes everything. From that day on you have another label – wife, mother, sister, husband, father, brother and… cancer patient.

A diagnosis of cancer can keep people locked in a process that is akin to being on a conveyor belt. The focus on saving life is understandable but also tends to make the whole experience very negative. Anxiety and fear are like the sabre tooth tiger outside our cave – they increase cortisol in the body, promote the fight or flight response and get in the way of healing.

The myth is that we are powerless to change the course of the disease and that only immediate medical intervention will 'save' us. I believe that medical treatment is essential to buy us time to rethink our lives and decide what is needed for healing in our whole life – mind, body and spirit.

The focus of cancer treatment is to remove the tumour (or shrink it, at least) and to remove all vestiges of cancer from the body in the hope that metastasis or a recurrence never happens. This is quite right.

However, if the focus is only on quantity of life, it can increase fear and bring about a sense of failure if the cancer does return.

Even when you are cancer-free you are labelled a 'cancer survivor' – a much-desired outcome by the health system as it validates the investment governments make in current treatment protocols. Maybe we are survivors of 'life' and cancer is just another aspect of life on a toxic planet?

There seems to be a bubble of negativity around illness in the 21st century when we have the best medical system since time began. Perhaps we can embrace the hope that medical science brings, support treatment with medically proven benefits of CM and replace the bubble of negativity and fear with peace.

## The type of cancer should not matter

As our medical treatments evolve and improve, more of us live well with cancer in our past and the experience of diagnosis and treatment becomes part of our story. When we share the memory, we dilute the trauma, validate the suffering and fear and affirm our connection as people who have had cancer. I have felt the catharsis of this process and feel deeply grateful to those who have listened while I tell my story.

I think this is why the breast cancer movement is so strong. I don't deny the benefits of women rallying to talk about the pain of breast cancer. I do think we can be much more inclusive. If you have cancer, regardless of where in your body it is located, you need all the compassionate understanding you can find. Life with cancer isn't about being worthy, young, beautiful or having small children. Life with cancer sucks, and treatment is an endurance test – physically, emotionally and spiritually.

We are all mutilated in some way. For a time, we are controlled by fear and uncertainty, feeling vulnerable as we are given complex information and pressured into making decisions.

There is still implied shame or blame around certain cancers – for example, lung cancer means you smoked, cervical cancer means you were promiscuous, bowel cancer means you didn't eat properly. Myths abound, yet none have been proven to be entirely or even partially true.

Everyone diagnosed with cancer longs to be loved, held in compassionate arms and understood, whichever organ has succumbed to cancer.

Distinctions drawn between beautiful young breasts removed versus aging bones with blood cancer is a commercially driven distinction that thousands of people buy into every day until they have a loved one who missed out on the 'glamour' that sometimes surrounds breast cancer and must find their way through the minefield of cancer treatment alone.

## The journey and the battle

There is much to say about the cancer 'journey'. We change the language around fear and suffering, we trivialise it. Even death has become 'passing'. In the 20 years of 'hanging out' with folk on the edge of life, I have found them to be honest, straight talkers. Few need to soften the language around their experience of cancer or death.

Cancer is not a journey with travel brochures. It is a confronting experience littered with scientific jargon, floating on a sea of emotions that highlight all the parts of your life that need healing, change or something more than you have been able to give yourself, up until now.

The cancer 'battle' in our own body is also a common analogy. It can certainly feel like a battle – to endure treatment, to recover your mind and body and to live to tell the tale. But that is not the most helpful way to think about cancer. Why would you imagine that your trillions of healthy cells were 'battling' cancer cells in a fight to the death? At diagnosis, most patients have a tumour that is smaller than a fist. Why not imagine that your cancer cells are surrounded by trillions of healthy cells doing their very best to contain and reduce the cancer cells?

If we don't win the battle, we become a 'loser', and if we don't die on time, are we a 'winner'? Some side effects of treatment last a lifetime.

> I had a client who had breast cancer many years ago when the best-known treatment was radiation. I saw her recently when she was dying because of 'fibrosing lungs' caused by radiation a lifetime ago. Her poignant comment, 'All I ever did was what they told me to do.' Her sense of injustice grew over the years out of her feeling that treatment was 'done' to her, leaving her to battle years of breathlessness alone.

We all need to know the long- and short-term consequences of the treatment we are offered and dispel the myth that we won't understand. The breathlessness appeared to be her battle, but the sense of injustice stole her peace every day of her life.

When do healing and self-care become a battle? Maybe when treatment begins?

Isolation from the flow of life and abandonment by family and friends are most often part of any illness, but with cancer, it can feel like a battle. Diseases sap our energy and our sense of humour, we sleep a lot and we move slowly through our days. I have worked with many clients who use a week's worth of energy just to come for a massage.

Life truly does go on without us. This can be very confronting when we look our own mortality in the eye and feel abandoned. Partners, family and friends get worn out.

> On the cancer programs at QFL, I had the privilege of running the small group session with partners and loved ones who accompanied folk with cancer to the program. It was a revelation to hear their stories. Stories of loneliness and solitude while the sick person slept, fear of the future without their soulmate, fear of telling children that their mother had died, loss of friends because they could no longer leave the house and so much more. This is all part of the 'battle' that surrounds a person with cancer. It is never just the person with the diagnosis, it is everyone who loves them – their family, friends and community.

## Cancer and suffering

There are of course many people who cling to the 'bad old days' of cancer treatment and look at you with 'coffin eyes' if a cancer diagnosis is even suspected, let alone confirmed. That look of hopelessness is a very challenging experience for two reasons. Firstly, it assumes the worst and secondly, it projects the fear of the other onto the friend or loved one with the diagnosis. The look is usually followed by the most frightening and horrendous cancer story imaginable. An attempt at empathy?

The myth that is part of the 'coffin eye' response is, 'If you have cancer you have to feel bad.' Yes, cancer treatment isn't a walk in the park, but the side effects can be made more manageable wiith the right kind of massage(OM), exercise, meditation and, at times, medication. I'm amazed that we need medical research to validate this simple compassionate approach to cancer care.

> When my mum was in aged care at the end of her life, I arrived to find her sitting on the toilet in tears. She had misjudged her

# TOUCHING CANCER

> timing and there was a 'clean up' needed. I set about wiping her tears and we laughed about the changes that life brings. In my childhood, she changed my nappies! The young carer eventually came in to help us. Before she left the room, she said, 'Where did you learn to care for the elderly?' I responded, 'At my mother's knee'.

Cleaning folk of any age and preserving dignity is all part of life, part of the human condition. In sickness or in old age we don't have to 'feel bad' about ourselves, even if pain is a constant companion or our body is letting us down.

I have always spent a lot of time talking to OM therapists about their behaviour around 'coffin eyes' and the 'feel bad' attitude as it undermines the confidence of the person with cancer. It is a 'put down' that each therapist must work out how to manage in any situation. If they open their minds and hearts, their clients will teach them. Every sick person was once well, every old person was once young.

I have had clients who were worried that their chemo wasn't working because they didn't feel bad enough and the client who had a double mastectomy and didn't need any further treatment but insisted on a course of radiation 'just in case' and, in her words, she needed to 'suffer to feel like the cancer was gone'. We are a weird mob indeed.

> How you feel matters. Whether we live or die from our cancer, let's do it well. Let's tune in to our every thought and feeling, act on the positive and explore the not so positive until we know ourselves better than we ever imagined possible. An interesting way to live and die, eh?

# 5.

# Fundamentals of Oncology Massage

Now that we've talked about the science and the power of compassionate touch and debunked a few myths about cancer and massage, it's time to dive into OM itself and the courses that evolved from MC&M. Again, I need to stress that this is my story of the early days of developing the courses. Many people were involved later on and OM quite rightly developed a life of its own.

During the introduction to OM1, I was heard to say to students, 'I wish I had a microchip that I could download into your brain and THEN we could start talking about massaging very sick people.' There is quite a bit of medical and scientific understanding that supports a skilled and safe oncology massage. How could I bundle so much information into a three-day OM training program?

## Why is specialised training even necessary?

The typical massage school curriculum is all about musculoskeletal techniques, particularly deep tissue friction. However, these are not suitable techniques for massaging clients with systemic diseases. When the massage is painful, cancer treatment side effects increase, heart rate increases, blood pressure goes up, blood vessels constrict – these are the body's self-defence responses to pain.

If a person with cancer has a deep massage, they often develop flu symptoms that last for a few days. This experience leads to laying down a cell memory that communicates the message of 'massage equals pain'. People aren't silly; they rarely endure suffering from deep tissue massage and willingly come back for more. Often patients don't speak up (cancer patients are known anecdotally for their accommodating personalities) and they just avoid massage altogether.

With OM and other light touch techniques, the approach is completely different. Yes, the client still lies on the massage table and receives strokes to their body. But the strokes themselves are not as important as the way in which they are delivered – light (but not too light), nurturing, mindful, with the whole hand – and the client's trust that the therapist understands what their body is going through and will massage them safely. For clients to be able to surrender to relaxation, the environment needs to be like a bubble of calm and peace. Believe me, this can be challenging, but it is possible even in a busy hospital ward!

Over all the years I have worked with massage therapists aspiring to work with medically challenged clients, the most common worry they mention is 'if they might hurt the client'. Teaching people how to massage safely is integral to OM courses.

## Getting the word out

Twenty years ago, when OM was on the very edge of the massage community's imagining, I couldn't think where to begin to explain what I had experienced in my work with very sick clients. I relied on the resources coming out of MSKCC in New York, The Bristol Clinic in the UK, M.D. Anderson Clinic in Texas and, in time, S4OM.

It is very fashionable to have an 'elevator' speech about your product – a 60 to 90-second short and sweet summary. In 2000, this was a real challenge for me as I had so much to say! I found my 'elevator' talk by writing articles for anyone who would publish my papers. As I grew in confidence, speaking invitations came my way.

In 2007, the Australian Naturopathic Practitioners' Association (ANPA) awarded me the Professional Excellence Award in Journalism for an article about OM as a conduit for other complementary modalities to support advances in cancer treatment and quality of life in survivorship.

I watched closely the development of S4OM and OM training in North America and England. MSKCC and MD Anderson published consistently excellent papers and the Society for Integrative Oncology (SIO – a medical association) was established in 2007. I realised that with Australia's smaller population and even smaller CM community, we have a great advantage over our bigger cousins, and an opportunity to regulate the level of training that is needed before a therapist can work in a hospital or medical practice.

## Reaching for the sky

I believed from the beginning that it was vital to develop OM nationally and that the Australian Skills Quality Authority (ASQA), which governs massage training, was the stepping stone to acceptance by the medical community. I hoped that, if it was assessed by the highest standards available, our training could help OM become part of mainstream medical services. ASQA accredited courses for dental nurses and paramedics lead the way. Funding to train suitably qualified massage therapists in oncology massage would be found, because of better patient outcomes. Right?

When I first wrote MC&M and then the OM1 and OM2 training programs, I imagined that if I made them scientifically 'tight' enough, accrediting massage associations would support me in demanding that only therapists who had completed specialised OM training would get jobs in medical services, if and when jobs became available.

I chose to stay with the principles established by Gayle MacDonald and Tracy Walton when I started teaching OM in Australia. My idea was to support an internationally standardised training program that could be relied on globally. Our medical system needs certainty and consistency. Our massage community needs regulation and clear guidelines. Our clients need to be massaged safely.

I insisted that only therapists with at least two years' experience would be accepted onto OM2 programs. Through my interactions with massage schools, I noticed that after two years, many therapists were very self-aware and looking for a speciality. They knew what healthy people 'felt' like and I could expand their understanding of pathophysiology and how to treat clients with systemic diseases. However, considering that on average therapists only stay in the massage world for three years, this was a big ask!

I believed that the first OM therapists in Australia had to be exceptional communicators, willing to learn the science, be the equal of an allied health professional, comfortable with writing to their local GP or oncologist, and able to run a highly professional clinic. I charged more than any other massage training course in Australia at the time. My thinking was that I only wanted therapists who had a proven ability to earn a living. Only the best and most committed massage professionals got to hang my OM2 certificate on their walls!

Most therapists who enrolled were kind-hearted and had skilled hands, and I knew them all personally. At times I didn't allow therapists to proceed to OM2, mainly because their literacy and business skills were lacking, or they held confronting views about CM in relation to medical science. The towels and linen that students brought to the training sessions were always an indicator of their clinic standards. Some students brought threadbare linen and looked very casual indeed. If things didn't change naturally over the three days on MC&M or OM1, I embarked on a tricky conversation about professional standards and hygiene. In the early 2000s, associations didn't have any guidelines for washing linen, but after my motherly talk a satisfactory outcome generally followed!

## Coming back down to earth

Of course, my initial expectations were far too high, so I had to compromise a little here and there. I advertised that student therapists would learn the science of cancer, how cancer developed and spread, how chemotherapy and radiotherapy treatment worked and the emotional challenges of the cancer diagnosis and survivorship. An early teacher was unwilling to explain the science, especially epigenetics and fascial function. Subsequent teachers did a fabulous job of this, but in the early days I was flummoxed by how to do it by myself! I made a DVD with technical expertise from a dear friend, which is still used.

An abundance of thinking and imagining had to happen before I printed the first training manual. Then, as reality unfolded, changes had to be continually written into the paperwork. For a scatterbrain like me, this was a nightmare!

Developing the business side of transition from MC&M to OM1 and OM2 was beyond my skill set so I concentrated on S4OM's approval and fine-tuning the course content. S4OM and local massage associations approved my expanded course content immediately and in 2008 OM1 and OM2 were off and running.

## Getting paid

Volunteer massage therapists in medical settings do a fantastic job. But I knew that if trained OM therapists volunteered, they would never gain acceptance onto the wards or into outpatient clinics, have access to patient files or work collaboratively with doctors and nurses. OM therapists need to be paid a fair and reasonable salary for the support they offer medical staff and the comfort they provide to patients.

Against my advice, many early students started working as volunteers in their local hospitals. Not one, not even a talented OM teacher, was ever employed by the hospital in which they volunteered. If you start as a volunteer, you will be stuck with that label. Why would any employer pay for something that they are already getting for free?

> In the very early days, Sir Charles Gairdner Hospital in Perth boasted that they had a large team of volunteers who did OM. The recruiting was pitched at graduating massage students, and they were encouraged to join the volunteer team and get valuable experience before they went out to establish their own clinics.
>
> The founder of this service, a terrific doctor, sat on the NSW Cancer Institute committee at the same time as I did. I would 'front' him at every opportunity, explaining my concerns. I even met with the director of the service in Perth and his longest-serving volunteer massage therapist. At this meeting, I asked the experienced OM therapist, 'If your wife came home tomorrow and said she was ready to retire and travel, would you go or stay to volunteer at the hospital?' He said he would go travelling with his wife. Point taken. With volunteers, the OM service does not retain expertise that will establish the modality as an integrative service. Also, they were bringing naive therapists into complex situations. Do we put a newly graduated nurse into ICU without intensive training and constant supervision?

Massage therapy education is not government-subsidised in any way. Massage school is expensive and annual professional development courses (like OM) are required for recognition by accrediting associations. OM therapists pay a lot for their training. We can make a reasonable living and we won't get rich. If we aren't massaging, we aren't getting paid.

From the early courses, I found likeminded therapists with exceptional skills. One had left a long career in banking to become a massage therapist, another had managed budgets and staff in retail and two of the Sydney therapists had run a successful massage practice together for over 10 years. They will always hold a treasured place in my heart.

OM teachers, the open-hearted women and one very special man, taught and mentored aspiring OM therapists around the country and developed connections with GPs and outpatient cancer clinics in each state and territory.

## OM1 – covering the fundamentals

### Energy and emotions

The first concept covered was the importance of totally focusing on the client for the whole massage, using Gayle MacDonald's pity versus compassion practice (Chapter 3). One student placed their hands on another's shoulders. Firstly, they were asked to think with pity, 'You poor thing, you are so sick', before removing their hands. The student replaced their hands and thought with compassion: 'You can do this,' and, 'I'm here to support you.' They removed their hands and asked for feedback from the other person. This experience is profound because what we think and feel changes what the other feels. Students were generally amazed that they could really feel the difference between pity and support.

We also demonstrated 'energy'. If you hold your palms about five centimetres apart and concentrate, you can feel heat. This is your own energy (chi) and this is what clients feel when we massage. The sensation comes and goes. I cannot 'make' this heat happen when I'm massaging; it just does. In the first practical session, the students practised on each other, feeling changes in skin temperature and noticing their own chi – manifested as 'hand heat'.

### Inching forward

Remedial massage therapists often move quickly to assess muscles early in the treatment, allowing time to return to the tight bits and work more deeply. One of the first lessons in OM is to slow down. It's important to breathe with the client, try to meet their pace of life. When we are sick it feels like the world and everything in it is whizzing past us.

Even applying lotion or oil is a careful, nurturing process that assures the client that you are going to work mindfully with the parts of their body needing to relax and let go. This 'lotioning' builds trust and sets up the internal response in the client. The entire massage needs to embody this beginning, with slow, rhythmic movements that suit the client's physical and emotional state at that time. We hope that our client feels that we are 'inching (them) forward' with care and compassion.

Sometimes inching forward means stopping the massage. Therapists are taught that if they ever encounter an area of the body that is hot, red, tender or swollen, they must stop the massage immediately. They could have discovered an infection, blood clot or undetected inflammation like cellulitis. I reassured students who were worried that they would miss a contraindication by telling them that in my experience, contraindications are very obvious.

> I have established a wide circle of allied health professionals and I work at communicating with a client's GP and oncologist where possible. These like-minded professionals know my work

and take my referrals seriously. On one occasion, I took a client with a deep vein thrombosis (DVT) straight to hospital. We were both treated with respect, gratitude for quick action and acknowledgement of my professionalism.

## Pressure, site, position

The OM mantra – pressure, site, position – is the key element of our teaching. The mantra was repeated many times during the course and discussion encouraged around the concepts, all helping to carry home the message.

### Pressure

The small body of medical research and a mountain of observational and anecdotal evidence consistently report that light pressure massage in a peaceful environment activates the relaxation response and creates positive changes in our bodies.

Tracy Walton has a wonderful diagram describing appropriate pressures during an OM and she generously allowed me to include it in the teaching manual.[17]

- Level 1 – Lightly lotioning the skin.
- Level 2 – Firmer lotioning of the skin so the skin caresses the fascia.
- Level 3 – Slightly increasing the pressure so that the fascia caresses the muscle.

And that is it. Not deeper… ever!

As the pressure goes from one to three, a slight ripple of skin develops in front of the leading hand. This ripple is swept along with gentle

---

[17] https://www.tracywalton.com/wp-content/uploads/2015/04/Walton-Massage-Therapy-Pressure-Scale-for-WEBSITE.pdf

care until it merges with an area where there is a natural change in direction, such as the base of the back or the armpit.

I demonstrated pressure by 'sharing' the legs of the therapist on the table. The student applied oil to one leg and I did the same to the other. The person on the table gave us feedback, ensuring that our pressure was the same. I called out, 'One, two or three,' until the receiver was satisfied that our pressure consistently matched.

The rhythm of an OM means that the therapist must learn to hold themselves differently. During a remedial massage, the therapist uses their weight to apply pressure to the tight muscles of the client, relaxing into the transfer of pressure from time to time. During an OM, the therapist must carry their own weight all the time, carefully noting if the fascia beneath the skin is being compressed and backing off while maintaining a rhythm.

*Site*
The site that is massaged depends completely on what is happening for the client at that time. We don't massage the area of the body where there is a contraindication like lymphedema, a new scar, skin lesions or inflammation of any kind. Therapists also learn how to deal with common devices such as ports, stomas and cannulas. I have managed to find somewhere to massage or hold even when a person is in ICU or teetering on the edge of life.

> Gayle's in-hospital course in Portland, Oregon, was the adventure of a lifetime. So many stories, but what I'd like to share is an experience that changed what I taught in my programs.
>
> In the 39-bed bone marrow transplant unit, I was awaiting allocation to a patient. I heard a doctor ask Gayle if anyone in the group was familiar with infection control and she looked straight at me. My St Vincent's experience was coming in handy

in my new OM world. I was briefed about a patient who had 'graft versus host' syndrome. He had been in the same room for seven months and, among other things, had developed a highly contagious lung infection.

I put on PPE and gently pushed on the closed door. The patient had a drip in his arm and on his legs were two knee-high fluid pumps emitting a high-pitched squeal. The TV was blaring, and his wife sat in the corner in her PPE, reading a book. I asked if he would like a back rub and he refused. My response was, 'I've come all the way from Australia just to massage you!' This was rewarded with a grin. I started looking for somewhere to 'touch' safely. The only place I could see was his thigh. He reluctantly agreed to some lotion on his dry and scaly legs.

For 10 short minutes, I applied lotion to his left thigh, then asked if I could do the same on the right leg? He agreed. Ten minutes later, I quietly left the room. Removing the PPE, I felt grateful for the peace and quiet of the corridor.

The next day, I donned the PPE again and slipped into the room. This time he rolled over so I could put my 'lovely oil' onto his upper back and shoulders. I massaged his back and head, the 12 inches of both thighs and his hands. I repeated this pattern daily until the last day of the program. Interestingly, the TV became quieter and his wife more engaged.

At the post-course debrief, I was told that my reluctant patient's mood had lifted so much that he had agreed to leave his room for the first time in over seven months to do rehabilitation exercises.

When I came home, I upgraded the teaching manual to include the 'leg sequence', which was later formalised by one of the teachers.

*Position*

In order to relax, clients need to feel comfortable. If people are very ill, they cannot lie in certain positions (especially face down), so the OM needs modification to massage the areas that are accessible. Most people can sit somehow, so the legs can be gently massaged, and arms and neck can often be included. We ask people, 'What position do you sleep in?' When sick people are comfortable, they sleep, so that position is usually the one we go with. Side lying, with a pillow between the knees, feels nurturing and comfortable for many clients, particularly with warm covers and a smaller pillow to cuddle!

**The science**

Then it was time to leap into cell theory and the science of cancer (see Chapter 2).

Many students had fears left over from high school about learning science or relied on outdated information. Starting from the science of 'now', like epigenetics and cell membrane function, I opened up wonderful conversations. I relished the many 'lightbulb' moments of adult learning.

Most therapists knew about cancer, such as 'staging' of a tumour, as it is talked about in families, and clients remember details to write on medical intake forms. Clients often use the time with an OM therapist to talk about the emotional rollercoaster they have been on since they felt unwell or found a lump. They often retell the story of how they were given the news that they had advanced cancer and what it felt like to hear 'stage IV', or they were told to 'go home and get their affairs in order'.

**Cancer treatments**

I taught therapists how cancer treatments might affect clients and how the massage plan changes as a result. All cancer treatments have come a long way in the past 20 years; however, the side effects can still be debilitating, and the skills and understanding of an OM therapist can improve quality of life for most clients.

*Chemotherapy*
Chemotherapy (chemo) drugs are designed to kill all fast-growing cells, healthy or cancerous. Most fast-growing cells are in the gastrointestinal tract, so cancer patients are often very sick while the drug cycles through the active phase and they reach their lowest point (called the nadir) mid-cycle. After this low point, the body begins to recover and clients gradually feel better each day until their next dose of chemotherapy.

The chemotherapy cycle affects the role of OM for the client. Some clients book a massage on the day before chemo as they don't want to leave home until they are over the worst of the side effects. Some clients book a massage at their lowest point, as they feel better immediately after the OM. Compassion is the key to working with people with cancer or in cancer treatment. Many clients need to change their mind on the day of the massage. I took many a phone call saying, 'I can't come today, I'll call when I can to rebook'.

> *I told the students that I found this difficult at first, as my livelihood depended on paying clients. First, I decided to limit the number of cancer clients in my working week to lessen the financial impact, then I decided to think differently. If a client cancelled at short notice (too late to invite another client to fill the space) it was just God giving me more free time that I didn't know I needed.*

There are many considerations for a client having chemo, which can feel overwhelming at first but become routine with practice:

- clients might have flu-like symptoms due to low white blood cell counts;
- if the white blood cell count is low, then strict hygiene is vital as the client's immune system is suppressed;

- the client might bruise easily due to low platelets in the blood;
- the skin could be fragile or sensitive due to nerve damage;
- there might be an indwelling central line for administering chemotherapy;
- there might be nausea for a variety of reasons; and
- the client may be feeling anxious, depressed or traumatised.

The list is extensive and OM teachers have insights and stories to teach their students about the best OM practice to provide for clients.

### Radiotherapy

Radiotherapy has been around for over a century and gradual refinements have relied on breakthroughs in technology.

> I became aware of radiology in 1966, when my best friend from school took a job at St Vincent's Hospital in the Radiotherapy Department. We were apprentices together and drove from the Western suburbs to inner Sydney each morning in our white uniforms to learn a very hands-on kind of medical science. We thought we were 'it and a bit'!

Once a client has been treated with radiation, there are more 'safe touch' considerations:

- The area that has been treated is marked out with little black dots that are tattooed on the skin – a lifetime reminder. This area is usually red and must not be touched.
- Another area to be mindful of is the 'exit' burn. As radiation techniques have improved this side effect is much better managed but in the early days of teaching OM it was really important to remember as it was usually on the back – the very place the client generally wants a massage.

- A vital part of patient safety is to look carefully at the patient's body, front and back, and only touch with compassion and gentleness where all is well.
- The lotion or oil must be medically approved – radiation burns stay hot long after the machine has finished delivering treatment and oil moves along creases and wrinkles towards the 'hot' areas of the body.
- Other major side effects of radiation include fatigue and depression – even more reason to go slowly and carefully and build trust so the client can truly relax.

Radiation departments used to be located in the basement of the hospital, sombre places that could leave patients feeling isolated during treatment. Some folk faced the experience with humour, while others just endured. Newer hospitals provide a more inviting environment, yet it is still a daunting procedure to endure.

> Folk with head and neck tumours have a mask moulded to their features and then the mask is screwed to the bench they lie on for treatment, to immobilise the head and ensure the treatment area is accurate. This process is traumatic for both the patient and the technician. Some years ago, I began a very positive discussion with a rural radiologist in a hospital connected to Austin Health and we planned to do research based on OML's leg massage technique (anecdotally known to reduce anxiety) done while the mask was being made and fitted. It was progressing well, and grant proposals were written. When the co-researcher took long service leave, her replacement stopped the project as it was too time-consuming to be completed during her work hours and no one else was prepared to do it in their own time (as we had done from the beginning of the project!). Despite this, it remains a very worthwhile research project.

*Surgery*
Surgery is a skilful tool to remove cancer, at the least to de-bulk the tumour and relieve symptoms, at best to excise all the margins and effect a cure. After surgery that did not remove all the tumour or couldn't remove any of it due to location (like brain, bone or bloodstream, the use of chemotherapy (like hormone or immunomodulatory therapy) or radiation is an option for many people.

> Chris' prostate surgery left an inaccessible lymph node behind. Radiation was not an option as the node was too mobile and he was offered hormone therapy that went very well. He is living well, disease-free and any recurrence of the tumour will be detected by a simple, cost effective, regular blood test. If the PSA (prostate specific antigen) titre rises he can have more hormone treatment. I hope Chris will be one of the majority of men with prostate cancer who will die 'with it' not 'of it'.

Not surprisingly, post-operative massage also has a few rules:

- If the scar isn't healed, the therapist must stay away from the quadrant of the body affected by the surgery.
- After six to eight weeks, if healing is healthy, gentle scar work can begin.
- If the operated area is not ready to be massaged then there are many other parts of the body that can be – such as hands, feet or head. Skilful oncology massage anywhere on the body can elicit the relaxation response to support healing.

*Times are changing*
As further medical advances are made, there are many more cancer treatment options available, including immunomodulatory therapy, more personalised chemotherapy regimens and CT or PET scan guided radiation. However, the fundamental principles of inching forward,

and pressure, site, position, remain essential. In my experience, every contact with a client experiencing cancer or cancer treatment must be *full* of compassion. Clients must be touched gently with the therapist's words, attitude and, most importantly, skilled hands.

Also, over my career in science and now in massage, it is interesting to observe how the levels of intervention have slowly increased.

> An elderly client (83 when we started) came to my home weekly in 1999 while I was learning massage and Bowen therapy. She let me learn on her, for which I am grateful. She kept me on track with her candid assessment of my progress. She saved $5 notes from her weekly shopping and I got them all (usually $15).
>
> After many weeks of gentle remedial massage, I asked if I could try BT. The first time I did a BT treatment, she went home happy then rang me half an hour later saying, 'The pain is back.' 'What pain?' 'The pain I had when I had transverse colon cancer.' This information was not on her intake form!
>
> At age 50, she had undergone major surgery to remove a very large tumour in her bowel. After the surgery, her take home message from her wise surgeon was, 'Go home and take as good care of yourself as you do of your family and you will be fine.' There was no further medical intervention offered or expected by the patient. She lived well and went on to reach a century. The 'pain' never returned, and she continued to come to me for BT, assess my progress and give feedback, whether requested or not!

Public opinion and times have changed.

> Just a few years ago, a colleague in her early 60s had both breasts removed due to a slow growing breast tumour. The surgeon was happy he had removed all the cancer and he could preserve all the lymph nodes. No further treatment was required, and the prognosis was excellent. This client demanded chemotherapy or radiation. She told me, 'I haven't been sick enough to be cured'.

### Lymphatics

One final section of theory was needed for therapists to understand the 'watersheds' of the lymphatic system. I teach that OM is safe massage for people with compromised lymph nodes, but it is not lymphatic drainage.

All massage moves fluid within our bodies, and I believe that every tactile therapist must understand how the body processes lymphatic fluid. Lymph nodes are found throughout the body and in higher numbers in the groin, armpits, neck and abdomen. Fascia creates a natural river directing lymph fluid towards the nodes ensuring that waste, like unwanted cells, is eliminated. The lymphatic system is like a passive blood system without a heart to pump the fluid, relying instead on our muscles to contract to move the fluid to the right place in the body. Lymph fluid empties into the bloodstream and is excreted via the kidneys and sometimes the large bowel.

Where the lymph fluid changes direction naturally is called a 'watershed' and, especially when very light touch is applied to the skin, lymph fluid can be directed around the 'watersheds' to help the body process it effectively.

This is a very big topic. Understanding 'watersheds' is critical to understanding safe massage for people with compromised lymph nodes (following surgery or radiation) and we devote several hours of OM training to this topic.

### *When do we offer massage?*

With all of these potential side effects of cancer treatment to consider, when do we offer a massage to a client with cancer or a history of cancer? This was always a huge question for the students.

In my experience, the best time for a massage is when the client asks for one! OM is so safe that it can be given anytime, as long as the client can relax enough to benefit. Some people decide it isn't right for them at all, saying, 'Don't touch me, I'm too frightened and fragile.'

> Another dear friend trusted me to massage her before and after her cancerous kidney was removed. The time between diagnosis and surgery is a very stressful time and I suggested that she try OM daily during that period. Her approach on the day of the surgery was a delight to witness. Her BP was normal, her mood calm and her belief in a successful operation inspired her surgical team.
>
> The kidney was successfully out and on day three she was in her private room. As gently as I could, working with her ability to move and position herself comfortably, I lotioned her back and lower legs while she drifted in and out of sleep. I visited her daily until she left hospital, always asking the question, 'Where would you like me to work today?' At home, I popped in every three to four days and she gave me permission to massage more and more of her body.
>
> 'This must be feeling good or she wouldn't allow it,' was my thought. It was exciting. At her six-week check-up with the surgeon, he commented how extremely well she was, given the extensive surgery. Her vitals were great. Her doctor asked what she had been doing in her six-week recovery. She answered, 'Regular massage,' and his reply was, 'That wouldn't do it.' Ho hum!

### Practise, practise, practise

Then came time for the therapists to practise OM techniques on each other. Students massaging each other was the best way for them to understand that 'less is more' – to back off and be gentle.

Gradually, they realised that the key to OM is activating the relaxation response. As they left OM1, I asked them to practise the techniques they had learned on healthy family members, re-read Gayle's *Medicine Hands* and Petrea's *Your Life Matters*, and think carefully about whether they wanted to work with very sick people. I gave them a list of online references and asked all my students to call or email if they wanted to discuss anything that cropped up for them.

OM 2 started six weeks later, and I rang therapists to check if they wanted to continue and if so, that they had done their homework reading.

I learnt by experience what I wrote into my MC&M/OM1 training course, and it was interesting to watch the teachers I trained write up all the information that didn't get onto the pages of the course manuals. From their observation of my teaching (it was different every time) came the teacher manuals. I am so grateful for this work because over time the teachers created student and teacher manuals second to none.

## Delving into the detail in OM2

When we gathered again for OM2, I revisited science and pressure, site, position and we discussed ideas that 'life' and reading had brought up based on the therapists' new understanding of massage and relaxation.

OM2 went into detail about how to put theory into practice.

In summary:

- Slow down, don't work on the muscles, lotion the skin and the soft fascia just below the skin.
- Minimise conversation with the client. Aim to bring peace and stillness to people who may be living a nightmare of fear and physical suffering.
- Drape towels or sheets carefully and gently – being tucked in and warm is very comforting.
- Warm the room so that taking clothes off does not create a temperature shock.
- Don't wear revealing tops – the last thing a post-breast operation client needs is to see your breasts.
- Don't rent a room that requires clients to climb a set of stairs.
- Ensure every piece of linen used in the massage is expertly cleaned and new looking – sick people need to feel valued and valuable.
- Take strict hygiene and infection control measures in the clinic, as many OM clients have weakened immune systems.
- Allow clients to position themselves where they are comfortable and do not rearrange them to suit your idea of 'straight'!

In OM2 we also discussed ways to take OM into the community, like starting a dialogue with local GPs or hospital cancer services, running information sessions for cancer support services and establishing supervision consults with local psychologists who understand the work.

### Intake process

The intake procedure was important to teach as the information alerts therapists to any contraindications, gives insight into the energy level of the client and begins a therapeutic relationship of trust. The skills of reflective listening were taught, although most students already had this skill.

Confidentiality is basic to trust and for folk in a traumatic situation is very important. Scope of practice is unique to this work too. Are you qualified to discuss nutrition or supplements, spa services or exercise, meditation or yoga? If not, then don't!

### Skin and scars

All massage therapists are taught in massage school that observing the skin is an important part of their job. Skin rashes, lumps, moles and freckles can be tricky, especially if the client has a history of cancer. Skin rashes are complex and have many causes. OM therapists need to understand how skin grows and sheds, as well as common diseases of the skin. I have massaged many clients with unusual skin blemishes and lumps. I avoid the area, I don't alarm the client and I ask them to see their doctor before they book another massage.

Managing complex scars is a gift to both the client and the therapist.

> A common story is that the patient has chosen a trans-flap operation where the abdominal fat or the latissimus dorsi muscle is moved subcutaneously up to the breast site, or an implant is inserted at the initial surgery to replace the removed breast. A complex healing process follows these procedures and there are scars, mostly under the skin and out of sight. I have seen astounding results with gentle fascial release techniques on complex subcutaneous scars. Pain relief is almost instant as the fascia relaxes and subcutaneous moisture begins to flow.

Bodies change shape all the time and what was a perfect join in the flesh at the time of the surgery might be misplaced after a year. Weight gain is not uncommon when treatment is over and a sense of health returns. OM2 has a session on advanced scar management that answers complex questions from the therapists who have been working with friends or family since they completed OM1. Complex scars are tricky to treat without the insights of the OM2 teaching. Once the skin scar is healed, deep tissue friction is usually applied to the scar by a physiotherapist, which is often painful. OM techniques are gentle and deeply effective.

### More science – of course!

My science lectures were pretty standard cell biology, but my lectures on safe touch were the opposite to massage school techniques. With all the body changes we see in oncology clients, we cannot follow a routine or pattern. Every client poses a new challenge and we can't become habitual in our approach.

Experienced therapists found it confronting and challenged me to ground my teaching in research, although unfortunately there was little to work with. Gayle MacDonald's *Medicine Hands,* in its third edition, is still the most comprehensive OM textbook today.

In OM2, we covered course material including the body's response to injury, how we age and adapt biologically and how we die. OM2 notes explored the medical fields of 'psycho-neuro-immunology' (PNI) and more on epigenetics, fascinating topics for OM students because they explain so much about who we are and how we think. There was also a lot more about safe massage for clients with compromised lymph nodes and lymphoedema, including when to refer clients to another health professional.

There was always lively discussion around spontaneous remission and the role of cancer support groups.

### Assessment

The OM2 practical sessions were about examining students on the skills we taught in OM1 and teaching scar massage, global release of fascia, breast massage and abdominal massage (to relieve constipation).

We spent time doing case studies with an element of role-playing. A plan was developed by the massage giver and brought to the teacher for checking to ensure all OM techniques had been considered. Interestingly, some therapists avoided certain areas of the body or the use of particular techniques. Often a conversation about science or beliefs at a critical time in the learning process, with a teacher close by, addressed these reservations.

All course content was examined through an 80-question multiple-choice exam. My first attempt at an exam was thought to be too tough so it has been modified by teachers over the years. It is still a good reflection of what is taught in OM1 and OM2 and includes general knowledge about common diseases.

The last part of OM2 was a practical session where the OM2 therapist gave a massage to a client with cancer or a history of cancer. This included a full intake process, treatment plan, supervised massage and time with the client after the massage. After all the clients had left, the teachers and student therapists sat in a circle and shared their experiences.

Where I would find and how I would manage 12 to 18 sick people every course never occurred to me until I was in the thick of it. It was a wonderfully stressful experience for teacher and students. I was setting my sights on excellence and trusting that folk with cancer would come for a free massage, and they did.

> I remember the teacher in Adelaide, a registered nurse (RN), running around the Royal Adelaide Hospital finding folk to massage and all the patients coming to the teaching room in their dressing gowns. What an exhausting day that was.

## The role of OM in cancer care

OM won't cure cancer. It won't fix it, change it or make it better. What OM can do is create a state of bliss and peace in the body that encourages space for healing. OM is about holistic care and improving quality of life. When we know that we are touched with compassion, thoughtfulness and without judgement, peace and deep relaxation moves our immune system towards healing chemistry.

This feeling is affected by the pressure, site and position of the contact that is the skill of the therapist. That is what OM is all about.

## Taking it home

At the end of the course, we all go back to our world as it was before we learnt OM. Nothing has changed, but the student has. The new OM therapists have learned that they must manage their emotions so that they can remain open-hearted and present-centred, leave judgement outside the treatment room and know when to refer the client to the right health professional for care.

Putting the principles of OM into clinical practice can be tricky. Most therapists have earned a living from remedial or Swedish massage, and they are emotionally geared to giving clients what they ask for – after all, that is what keeps clients coming back and paying the therapist's mortgage. It takes some people a while to trust the new techniques they have learned, and some never do.

The students also take home the teacher's phone number! OM training does not end when the course finishes. Each day, new OM therapists will potentially take on a client who has cancer or a history of cancer and they need to remember a lot of new facts from the course. A discussion with the OM teacher, with questions relating to a real situation, are moments of deep learning for the new OM therapist.

The follow-up mentoring was both a joy and a tricky endeavour, depending on the therapist's personality.

> I remember a phone call from a new OM therapist with over five years' experience in the remedial massage industry. She rang to alert me to a complaint from her client's GP. She (the therapist) had forgotten the 'gentle' rule, no 'inching forward' in this massage, and her client was badly bruised. She had low platelets. The GP gave me 'the rounds of the table' and threatened me with termination of my massage association membership and getting my course 'banned'. I managed to calm the GP by emailing her my training notes, the student's exam and assessment data and the MSKCC research paper. Phew! The therapist apologised, thanked me for speaking with her and even sent me a necklace as a gift.

Ongoing mentoring is essential.

### Keep inching forward
In the words of Deepak Chopra (1997):

*The body is not a mindless machine: the body and mind are one.*

This quote reminds me that every day is different for every person, and this is particularly true for clients with systemic disease. The phrase 'inching forward' is very important to bear in mind when an OM therapist has been seeing a client regularly. Each time we see a client, we assess them as if it is the first time. If the client wants a deeper massage, like they may have been offered last week, the therapist must explain why they are doing a gentle OM today. It is usually because there has been stress or a challenging event during the last few days. Sometimes it is because they are not as 'bright' as they were last week.

Gentle 'inching forward' accounts for the emotional pathway we all travel as we heal or die.

### *Remember self-care*

Working with people diagnosed with cancer or with a history of cancer is a specialist field, as we need to deal with our mortality every day. The need for therapists to model self-care for their clients is why Petrea's book *Your Life Matters* is so important for OM2 students.

It is commonly acknowledged that folk with cancer are 'lovely' people. We often hear, 'They don't deserve cancer, they're always there for everyone.' And it is true. Clients with a diagnosis of cancer are often 'imploders' as opposed to 'exploders' and are a delight to massage until you hear, time after time, that the cat is more important than they are. At that point, it becomes heartbreaking and likely to lead to a sorry end.

Often these same kind-hearted people are drawn to massage school and OM. It has been very important to include a lot of 'self-awareness' units in the OM programs. When I saw myself in others with cancer, I had the QFL teaching to sustain my inward journey. The nine years at QFL woke me up in many ways. I still got cancer. I still tend to put others ahead of my needs and need friends to remind me to give from my 'overflowing cup' rather than an 'empty bucket'. Habits accumulated and entrenched over a lifetime are hard to change.

### *Stay resilient*

Resilience is essential because integrating into the medical world requires a thick skin!

> I remember teaching in Queensland in 2005 at Bloomhill, an early cancer support centre funded by charity shops. The therapist who introduced me to the centre was a young woman whose huge heart, full of commitment, passion and patience,

> was a gift to OM for many years. Back then, she asked me to teach OM to the massage and nursing teams. The ten therapists were lively and interested in everything I had to say. The nurses observed rather than participated and I ran the course in the therapist's home as the conference room at Bloomhill was not made available.
>
> The therapists were already working part-time with cancer clients and had a wealth of experience to share. The team leader shared a little of her struggles with management and I quickly saw the 'line in the sand' between OM and what the supervising nurses expected of the massage therapists. The management wanted a standard, mechanical treatment without conversation (massage therapists are not qualified psychologists) and they were expected to use the same techniques every time, regardless of how the client presented. This was a totally unrealistic working environment and the employed therapists, knowing how much clients benefited from their work, turned themselves inside out to comply.

This group of therapists 'bubbled up' from many different backgrounds and they were a good representation of the women who wanted to study my course. Passion, commitment, compassion and a heartfelt desire to serve were common to them all. Especially in the early days, we were all learning together. The 'territory' challenges were so well hidden it often took us time to understand where the boundaries were actually being drawn. This was my training ground for what was to come.

Gentle-hearted massage therapists find it hard to be resilient in the face of intractable and powerful opposition. Some of the therapists I trained took up the OM challenge in their area, talking to GPs and hospital cancer centres. Some joined the OMT/OML teaching team. Others stopped offering OM and focused on other forms of massage that were more 'acceptable'. Even within the 'fold' of OML, most were reluctant to take on the integration challenge themselves. They wanted me to contact the hospital, write the article or somehow pave the way for them. Some, even when they were employed in the cancer facility and had great contacts, avoided the integration topic to avoid a personal rejection. Fair enough! It's no fun.

It became clear to me that running courses was no longer enough. I also needed to support the therapists, try to make it easier for them to find OM clients in their communities, and use my scientific and medical connections to smooth the path. Increasing numbers of people were relying on me for support, knowledge, facilitation, counselling and life coaching (before that was even a thing).

# 6.

# Taking OM into Hospitals

By 2007, OMT was well and truly up and running. My little business was beginning to take on a life of its own and I could feel the momentum growing. Why on earth did I feel the need to take the business to the next, even more challenging level? A few things happened that gave me a firm nudge in that direction.

In May 2007, I went to Germany for a month to attend the International Society of Bowen Therapists (ISBT) conference as a keynote speaker, together with John Coleman, a brilliant naturopath who had recovered from stage IV Parkinson's disease and multiple system atrophy. We also ran four OM courses in Germany and Austria. I found the time exciting and exhausting. My insights into massage for very sick people and my presentation of OM techniques were received very well. I could see that OM in Australia was a long way ahead of Germany at the time, in terms of understanding of massage for folk with systemic disease.

The ISBT therapists loved our courses and we enjoyed some fun times. The students were keen to host a meal or a beer with us. I felt like a rock star from Oz!

By 2008, OM1 and OM2 were recognised by the Society for Oncology Massage (S4OM) and endorsed by QFL, and we were certified to work safely and effectively with people diagnosed or with a history of cancer. I could see the benefits of the training and the confidence with which many therapists were treating clients in their communities, despite the challenges they faced. The work in Germany had started me thinking about the next logical step – taking OM into hospitals. I imagined OM therapists on staff in oncology wards, working alongside the medical staff and providing a valued service for patients undergoing active treatment or in palliative care.

Easier said than done! Introducing anything new to hospitals is no mean feat (pharmaceutical companies spend millions on research and development for just one new drug), and complementary therapies were considered unnecessary extras at the time. Little was known about massage training in general. Accredited massage associations were slowly establishing standards like a code of ethics but at the time, someone could open a massage business after completing a weekend course.

I was also already stretched pretty thinly! I was teaching every OM1 and OM2 program around Australia. I was still working at QFL to earn a living, training a handful of therapists how to teach my programs, seeing a diverse range of clients in my Canberra clinic, firing off articles to journals and magazines, studying more Bowen therapy with ISBT, presenting at conferences and expos, travelling to the US to attend conferences and undertake research, and talking about OM to anyone who would listen.

I felt honoured to be invited onto the NSW Cancer Institute (NSWCI) Committee to advise on OM. OM is being noticed at last, I cried.

But wait ... nothing actually changed. I attended three meetings in Sydney over the next two years, at my own expense. I looked around the board table and everyone but Eleanor had been paid to be there – by a hospital, a foundation, or a government department. If a massage therapist isn't massaging someone, they aren't earning a living. If a contract teacher isn't teaching someone, they aren't getting paid.

I would have donated my time willingly if I felt we were making progress. The content of the NSWCI meetings was always interesting, cutting edge and relevant but I never saw any of the research come to life or be understood by the general public. It felt like I was treading water. Petrea and I served on this committee for two years and then I decided to resign. At least it looked good on my CV! There were always so many competing responsibilities and I wanted to change the world with OM. I needed a clone, or maybe two.

## Thought leads to action

The move into hospitals really began when I was sought out by the CEO of a major Sydney private hospital, which had an excellent reputation for cancer treatment services. I had treated his partner at QFL and he was impressed by the positive changes. He opened the meeting saying, 'I want every patient in my hospital to have this treatment.' Gayle MacDonald was visiting Australia and came to the meeting with me, another fortuitous occurrence.

The CEO tasked the Director of Nursing (DON) with getting it underway – 'it' being a tactile service that would meet with the approval of specialist doctors and nurses who were the backbone of the hospital.

> As Gayle and I left the executive offices, we bumped into a hero of ours, Dr Catherine Hamlin. I encourage you to read her book,

*Hospital by the River*. She was a truly great Australian who spent a lifetime in Addis Ababa, Ethiopia, pioneering surgery to help any woman with a fistula caused by childbirth. Child marriage and the lack of midwife support leads to many young girls needing the surgery that Catherine and her husband pioneered. Catherine Hamlin changed the lives of countless young women and her work continues today – a legacy I greatly admire.

Gayle and I took this brief encounter with Catherine Hamlin as a 'wink from God' that we will never forget. We even imagined one day we might go to Catherine's hospital to teach OM and BT. It might still happen.

### An adventure in the US

Before I pursued the idea of taking OM into hospitals, I decided to do Gayle MacDonald's in-hospital training in Portland, Oregon. Within a few short weeks, I was flying to the US and lodging in Gayle's spare room. I hit the ground running, with a crash course in everything Gayle could think of that might prepare me for the road ahead. At Portland's St Vincent's Hospital, we saw a therapist lead a patient through a meditation during their radiation session. What a great idea!

The OM training was fantastic. The hospital was huge and the fellow students generous. They shared their experience of hospital volunteer massage services, as well as enlightening me about cultural norms. Buying coffee was my first hospital challenge and great fun with my Aussie accent!

Gayle's course covered all aspects of communication with hospital staff and patients. She made moving around the hospital environment an adventure, and even sent us on a treasure hunt. Gayle is a talented teacher and I just love her classes.

The key lesson was that all the OM services, at that time, were completed by OM therapists who were allowed into the hospital as volunteers. The one salaried hospital therapist I met was funded by Gayle from the money she received from students who took her courses. I was in the same position. Creating positions for salaried OM employees became my goal, but first, we needed to train them!

> I took a Nerf Gun home from America for my son. Getting the 'gun' through US airport security was tricky. I was surrounded by four burly men saying no, then a young chap joined the happy throng, immediately knew what I had in the box and I was waved through.

## Back home, the work begins

The Director of Nursing (DON) and I began meeting regularly (at a cost, as I had to fly to Sydney each time). The first obstacle was assembling the evidence. Thankfully, S4OM had excellent resources which I used to prepare information for the medical board meeting. OMT was still a one-woman operation, so I didn't have much time to put into it.

> I remember the first doctors' meeting I spoke at began with a late afternoon flight from Canberra, a slow trip by public transport across Sydney, attending a 7-9 pm meeting at the hospital, catching a taxi across Sydney and then the last plane to Melbourne. The next day I began teaching a large OM1 course. The venue was miles away from any shops and I needed to buy morning and afternoon teas for the students. I managed to locate a corner store, so I jogged out while the students

> practised the OM1 back massage (that I had just taught them) and I was back in time to serve morning tea. I taught Saturday, Sunday and Monday, then farewelled the OM1 students. On Monday night, I arrived home at 9 pm and took the rest of the week to recover.

The OM1 paperwork was relatively easy to complete as I just needed to record their attendance then print and send out certificates. Very few people didn't progress to OM2. After I ran an OM2, I had to mark the exams, print the certificates and post them around the country, then decide who I thought might be suitable to be invited to join the in-hospital training group, when or if it started.

### I finally asked for help!

I remember it was a Sunday night when I was faced with piles of computer work to keep track of this 'exploding' little business. I was in tears and totally overwhelmed, and Chris offered me this advice: 'Why don't you ask Kylie for help?'

Kylie, our eldest, was at home in Brisbane with her beautiful baby boy. Ideas come easily to Kylie, and she has dynamic business knowledge as well as being clever and very efficient. Would she be interested in my little business?

> I rang Kylie and outlined my dilemma, sent her the work I needed to complete and promised to pay for her time. She rang back within an hour. It had taken her just 23 minutes to complete what would have taken me three days. My relief was palpable, and I think Kylie was smiling in Brisbane.

We worked together for the next seven years. Kylie's skills eventually led to OMT evolving into OML, a registered charity, which is testimony to her business acumen, capacity for productivity and ambition. Her story is part of everything that happened since 2009 and I am filled with pride and gratitude for everything she brought to OM in Australia.

With Kylie managing the small group of skilled OM teachers in addition to the business side of OMT, I finally had time to develop a teacher workbook (this actually grew organically out of the notes the teachers-in-training took while I taught a class) and the energy to develop OM3 and OM4. The student notes and teaching documents took a long time to prepare, as I kept thinking of extra information that therapists might need to feel safe and capable in the presence of a GP or in a hospital.

### OM3 – preparing to work in a hospital

I have an abiding commitment to support medical services as well as cancer patients and wanted the overall goal of OM3 to be respectful integration. Sharing stories of how OM therapists could support medical staff was encouraging for students. OM therapists are not competitors with our medical colleagues; we complement what they offer people who are facing complex medical challenges.

I wanted my OM3 students to be accepted by the hospital. Initially, I gave a lecture to all the hospital physiotherapists and outlined our scope of practice and what outcomes medical research predicted. It was a long meeting and by the Q&A, there was a feeling that their 'territory' was being threatened by OM therapists. Lymphoedema management was the hottest topic, and I assured the group that we did safe massage for anyone with compromised lymph nodes and did not attempt lymphatic drainage unless specifically trained in that modality.

What evolved when we started training in the clinics and wards was truly special. The physios skilfully walked the patient down the corridors (getting each individual moving in the most appropriate way), the nurses brought medication or managed the routines of daily living, then the massage therapist brought peace and deep relaxation. The patient often slept for an hour or so after the massage and the nurses had more time to complete their paperwork or see to other patients. It was a win-win for all.

A focus of OM3 is adapting to hospital culture, as we needed to blend in seamlessly. During the course we lived on hospital grounds, used the café for lunch and coffee breaks, moved in and out of treatment areas and wards, and it felt so good. I knew we were in the right place at the right time. Teaching OM3 was a joy. The students were committed and the hospital opened its doors to us with kindness, even when I made little mistakes here and there.

We cooked our meals together in the evening and on occasion we danced after dinner or gave each other shoulder and foot massages. This was perfect for team-building, which is essential to this kind of work. I needed to know I was not alone in this heart-warming, and sometimes heartbreaking, work.

### Infection control and manual handling

Infection control and manual handling were taught early and often in the OM3 program as they are vital for hospital work. The first few groups of six therapists to do OM3 enjoyed the tuition of my dear friend, Greta, who had spent many years as an RN in aged care. Greta's lectures on hand hygiene and infection control were pitched at exactly the right level for my students, with every unit based on a 'watch me do it, then you do it' style. Initially, while Greta taught, I had time to ensure that I was ready to teach my sections. This was a great relief after teaching students and training teachers on my own for the past few years.

It was important to hear about injuries and mishaps from Greta's nursing experience. The rule for OM therapists was to contact the attending nurse and ask for help to position the patients if necessary. The most common request was for help to return the patient to bed so we could do a massage. Respecting nurses' skills helped to build a collaborative working atmosphere on the wards.

Therapists also learned how to put on and take off personal protective equipment (PPE) and use surgical gloves, which are mandatory when massaging patients with infections or actively receiving a chemotherapeutic infusion or in a barrier nursing situation.

A further consideration was how to dispense the massage lubricant so that it is safe from one patient to the next. In hospital, we dispense a small amount of organic, cold-pressed, almond oil into a pill-dispensing cup and put the cup into the rubbish at the end of the massage.

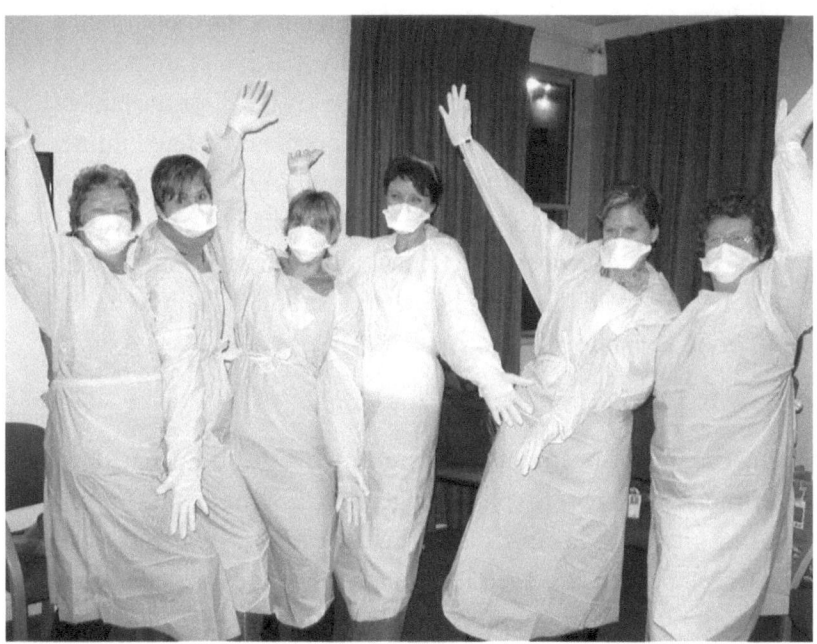

Practicing PPE in OM3.

### Communication is vital

Communication in the hospital is essential. Things like who to ask for clean towels. This might sound like a very simple request but in a busy ward, noisy and appearing chaotic, your request might distract the one person trying to remember a string of facts that need to be passed on immediately to a nearby colleague. Your simple request can use up precious time, annoy others and get you off on the wrong foot with the team you are hoping to support.

Getting a drink of water is relatively easy today, but ten years ago we had to know where the staff room was and then which cup we could use. Another difficult decision was knowing whether it was okay to enter a room.

> Folk in different uniforms trotted in and out of the room, closing the door behind them. Above the door was the number I had been given by the Nurse Unit Manager (NUM) for the patient in that room. I watched the flow of people for a few minutes and then knocked on the door and went in to find a complex procedure taking place and I was sternly asked to leave. Later, I asked the NUM what I should have done, to which she replied, 'You can't avoid moments like that, just don't take it to heart.' A good lesson to learn early.

Then, the announcements ringing out overhead. What did they *really* mean? What was code orange or red? We spent a lot of time ensuring that the therapists knew what was required of them if the announcement affected their location. Most nurses helped us in many ways with our settling in process.

I encouraged student therapists to ask the patient about the treatment they were on. It is not the therapists' job to understand every chemotherapy program, however our scope of practice does include understanding what our clients know about their treatment. This information is often written, and I have never been denied an information sheet in the chemo ward. Drug combinations often have similar side effects or none at all. Massage therapists need to know where the patient is in the treatment cycle as this often explains the way they present for a massage. OM therapists always wear gloves when massaging in the cancer wards. Communication is vital.

### Medical terminology

When I was doing Gayle's hospital course, a fellow student asked over a cup of coffee, 'Is myelin the same as myeloid?' The answer is no. Myelin is the tough sheath that protects our nerves. If the sheath develops plaques, we are diagnosed with multiple sclerosis (MS). Myeloid refers to the tissue that grows inside our bones and makes our blood. This made me realise the importance of OM therapists knowing as much medical terminology as possible.

I recommended a medical receptionist course, particularly for therapists practising in country towns. I often took phone calls from therapists stuck on pronunciation and we would have a good laugh.

The complex terminology of drugs and drug side effects is daunting for us all unless we are using it every day. Cancer drugs and side effects change rapidly and are highly specialised to treat a particular cancer. I expanded the dictionary of medical terminology in the OM1 and OM2 manuals to include the common terminology of hospital work.

Using correct terminology was very important because we had permission to write up our treatments in patient notes. Patient notes are legal documents and there are strict rules around how and where we could write our observations. We all felt that it was a privilege to have this door opened to OM and treated it accordingly.

## Understanding oncology treatments
### Radiation oncology

Understanding how the radiation oncology service worked was essential and the chief radiographer was amazingly forthcoming. She made time to come to our classes with DVDs in hand to teach us how the radiation machines worked and what services were available.

I described how things were going to flow when the students returned for OM4. When patients entered the radiation oncology unit, they went to a waiting room with activities like jigsaw puzzles and knitting. After treatment, they were directed to a quiet space that was peaceful and meditative. The hope was that in the peaceful room the patients focused on themselves and settled their thoughts and bodies before they went home. OM therapists were able to offer gentle foot and hand massage (without conversation), shoulder release or healing touch (resting hands on the head or back of the patient and feeling the warmth of chi) in this venue. The staff loved having us there and we soon became popular with the patients.

The stories of my experience also prepared the students, in a small way, for what was coming in OM4. My brachial therapy story was always keenly noted:

> Brachial therapy was a relatively new treatment for men with prostate cancer. The radiology machine fires rice-sized radioactive pellets into the walnut-sized prostate gland. Over hours or days, the radiation in the pellets destroys the cancerous tissue. This is painful and very quickly OM therapists were asked to offer shoulder release and foot massage for these patients. It was a privilege to offer safe touch to fearful men of all ages and I felt deep compassion for them all. Eyes often filled with tears after only a few minutes of gentle touch. It felt like we gave these strong capable men permission to weep, and there was much for them to weep about.

*Chemotherapy unit*
The Day Oncology Unit welcomed us too. There was a steady stream of patients at various stages of their treatment passing through this unit every day. The students wouldn't return to this area until OM4. I described what happened for the students and they took a lot of notes. The majority of our work was done while people sat in big comfortable armchairs receiving an infusion. Reactions to their treatment varied. I sometimes stepped back as the nurses moved in to manage the most severe reactions. On occasion, the 'code' team arrived and the patient was whisked away. In the main we gently worked with the patient's upper back, feet and arms, bringing comfort and peace during a frightening time.

In a small room off the main infusion area, patients underwent treatment for bladder cancer. They lay flat, then their bladder was infused with a chemotherapeutic drug and they turned every 15 minutes, back, left side, front, right side, for four hours. This was a great experience for my students as they had to adapt their OM to whatever area of the body presented itself every 15 minutes.

**Practical work**
OM3 had a series of case studies to help the students think about situations they may face in a hospital setting and reinforcing scope of practice principles.

The last day and a half of OM3 was focused on actually treating a client with cancer, recruiting 'volunteers' from the outpatient clinics. We always got the quota needed so every student had at least two real experiences. The conference area was transformed into a quiet space with dim lights and soft music. If an outpatient couldn't climb onto a massage table, we had reclining chairs, and this proved invaluable as it helped the students experience the real-life situation of hospital or home visits.

By the time OM3 started, all the students had heard my take on appropriate dress, especially necklines. New or near-new towels, freshly washed and aroma-free and the need for a vomit bowl that doesn't look like one, and your total attention, all the time, completed my list of 'must be aware of'.

Once the patient was up and dressed, the therapist escorted them to the seated area where a warm drink was offered, and the therapist ensured that they had assistance to get home. Next, I gathered the six students and they shared their client's story and their treatment plan, and reflected on the experience.

> A frail lady arrived with a very tall, well-dressed man. He told us that she was unsteady on her feet because she hadn't eaten since her last chemo three days ago. He was reluctant to leave her, and she insisted that he come back at the time we gave him (about 1.5 hours hence). Massage tables were all taken so I put her in a reclining chair. She was not happy with my decision and told me she was a language teacher, with all her faculties, in need of a 'proper' massage.
>
> Yes, you guessed it – I had chosen my least competent student for her massage, for a whole host of reasons that seem vague in my memory. I got busy supervising 16 therapists and didn't think about the 'very tall man' until he was standing before me telling me that his wife was just starting to eat her fourth sandwich while drinking her second cup of hot chocolate! Her seated massage had done the trick… how, I will never know, and my job is to be grateful. The therapist was stoked, and her skills improved markedly in her next supervised massage. It's all about confidence.

I remember how hard it was to tell a student that they were unsuitable to continue in the OM3 program. Everyone came to the program with an agenda of their own and most modified their expectations to facilitate a smooth, respectful transition into our OM community. Most difficult students were identified by the teachers of OM1 or OM2. However, some got through to OM3. One student came to our program to 'show the doctors and nurses' that CM was better than medicine. I think her long unwashed hair gave us a loophole in our contract with the hospital that saved our bacon. I refunded her course fees and then there were only five fee-paying students. Way below 'break even'! But I stuck to my guns.

## OM4 – a dream come true

Four weeks after OM3, we all came back to do OM4. What an adventure and a dream come true. OM4 focused on logistics. Where to be, at what time, to do what, to which patient?

Everyone arrived at the hospital on day one of OM4 with green polo shirts which had 'Oncology Massage Therapist' embroidered on the left breast pocket in bright orange, bearing a smile and shiny tied-back hair. We gathered in a café in the hospital and were greeted by other staff with, 'The leprechauns are back, they work miracles!'

The first day involved testing the students and filling all the gaps that had appeared in the weeks since OM3, like organising the session, seated massage intake, evaluation of the massage, outpatient intake, barrier nursing, writing patient notes and getting the patient consent form signed (a daunting three-page document prepared by hospital lawyers!).

It was impossible for me to supervise each student with my first group as there was only me. From then on there were two teachers to six students. Nurses and doctors are not so closely supervised. I think the hypervigilance was driven by the lack of understanding of massage training and highlighted the chasm between CM and mainstream medicine in Australia.

> I made a thoughtless mistake during the first course. I set up a portable massage table in the side room of the cancer ward and massaged a patient's son. I saw a need and I acted, as we did at QFL. The DON was furious with me as I was way outside of the contract guidelines. I feel embarrassed just remembering. The students gathered around me and got me through my tears, and we soldiered on… I was way too passionate about OM in the beginning.

The first six therapists to complete OM4 were outstanding women. They allowed me to muddle through with respect for me and they seemed to be aware of the many unknowns that confronted me. The routine was that the teacher accompanied the students on day one to ensure they got permission from a few patients to return at a set time to give them a massage. I split the students up into teams of two and I went with the first team and deposited them in the Day Infusion Unit, then I returned for another two students and took them to radiology and so it went, two by two. This process meant that four therapists had to wait for me to return to take two more out to another section of the hospital. This process had to change.

From day two, the student therapists were on their own, going to a different area in the hospital so eventually all the students got experience of every area. Then I 'hovered', thinking through all the things that could possibly go wrong – the things from 'left field', and then, finding that the student had found the best solution on their own, I breathed a sigh of relief. Every day was a physical exam on the wards and then I gave them a quiz to do overnight to ensure we had a paper trail of accountability. It was gruelling for us all.

By week's end, confidence was high, experience second to none in Australia and I could endorse every one of them in any job they found as an OM professional.

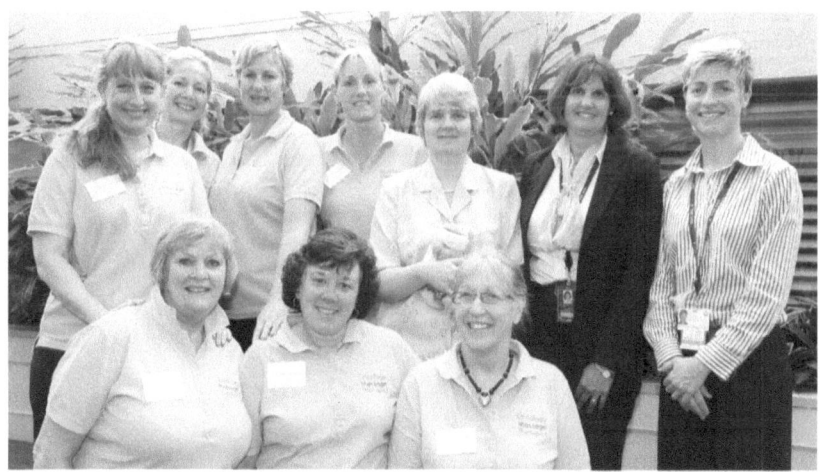

The first OM therapists in Australia Back row: Tania Shaw, CiCi Edwards, Lizzie Milligan, Tania Griffin, the cancer ward NUM, the DOM and the nurse educator. Front row: Christine Schipper, Gillian Desreaux, Eleanor Oyston c2009.

## The first hospital OM therapist is employed!

At the end of the first program, the DON asked me if any of the therapists in the course were suitable for employment by the hospital. I said, 'All of them.' Eventually, we talked around the needs and expectations of the hospital, and I named a therapist.

The full interview process for employment in the hospital started immediately and on the final day when the OM therapist was interviewed for the job she was asked to 'outline' a salary.

> I remember that day with a huge smile. Chris and I were in Melbourne at a dear friend's wedding and as we walked from the bus stop to the registry office, we were coaching the 'soon to be employed' therapist.

> 'Hold your ground,' 'You are one of seven internationally qualified OM therapists in Australia,' 'You have a busy clinic and you are making a solid living,' 'They need you more than you need them'. The first qualified OM therapist, with salaried employment in a hospital in Australia, was well paid. We fought for an equal wage with a senior nurse and in the end, it was only a few dollars short. In her role as OM therapist in a hospital, she was highly respected.

Within weeks, the nursing staff started to meet her as she arrived 'on the floor', directing her to a patient with abdominal pain from constipation, or a patient who was anxious or panicky. Her skilled massages were relied on and needed.

Within the first year as a hospital employee, the OM therapist presented a paper at the hospital-sponsored cancer conference. Six nursing staff from the ward where she worked sat in the front row of the conference room. When her talk was over, they gave her a standing ovation.

Nursing staff know the worth of having a qualified OM therapist on their team and unfortunately, the administration and accounting staff usually don't – until they do.

> During an in-ward OM massage of an elderly patient with advanced cancer, several administration staff came into the private room. The gathering around the bed caused the OM therapist to stop her massage and step to the side. The entourage had come to present a service award. The patient had been a senior employee in the hospital for several decades, whose colleagues and friends asked for feedback on hospital service and care. The patient said, 'The massage is the best thing that

> has happened to me since I was diagnosed.' Well, the massage therapist quickly rang me to share this wonderful endorsement. They will surely employ another OM therapist to support our 'lone ranger' on the cancer floor after this morning's blessing? Alas not.

At the beginning of the OM therapist's employment, we were told by the DON that she would be developing a team of OM therapists as the service would expand. Over the next two years there wasn't a single move to fulfil this promise and, after two years working alone, connecting deeply with very sick people, the therapist resigned. She was experiencing burnout.

The hospital offered her counselling with their chaplain which she took. It didn't take her long to realise that a chaplain 'holds hands' with death and distress while an OM therapist connects deeply with suffering and death. I have massaged legs that turned blue as the blood stopped flowing and the heart shut down. The patient was feeling blissful and connection in the final hours of life. I took my experience to supervision with a counsellor from the QFL team. OM therapists need to talk to other professionals who deeply understand their work and we need to work in a team.

For the two years of the OM therapist's hospital employment, I spoke with her while she drove home. We laughed and cried, and I began to feel a sense of guilt around setting up this service. What I had actually done was set my friend and colleague up to burn out. She was unsupported as there were no other massage therapists in her workplace, and it was heartbreaking to see this unfold. I was powerless to change a thing, so I worked harder to train therapists for hospital work, ready for the day that the medical model understood what we offered. Would our massage industry be ready?

This long sorry saga highlighted the need to keep OM therapists in hospital employment so that the professional expertise was not lost. Money alone was not the answer; she was paid well for her time massaging in the hospital. Isolation has only one cure – a team.

What I know from experience is that sustainable employment for a hospital OM therapist is seven hours a day, two days a week. Sessional consulting won't work no matter how skilled the therapist. I was told once by a very political doctor that she had run a successful CM private clinic on a sessional basis, and it would work in a hospital. She was wrong. Most multidisciplinary practices in Australia rent rooms to massage therapists, chiropractors and naturopaths, and her theory holds true (I have successfully worked in and run a clinical practice like this); hospitals and aged care facilities, however, are a totally different story. If a therapist is in the hospital for a day of work, then travelling time is unpaid work time, as it is for everyone else in the hospital's employ. If a patient is not in their room for some reason – X-ray, exercise class, family outing or sleeping – the therapist can move on to the next person within their hours of employment. If the therapist is sessional, they have to drive away and come back later. There are a lot of unpaid travel and waiting hours in the therapist's business.

The cost of running the in-hospital training in Sydney was becoming increasingly expensive. Every six months, the hire of the teaching room and the accommodation for students at the hospital increased. I imagine that the hospital looked at the amount per student OMT charged and they thought I was making a nice profit.

In the second year, I delayed signing the contract renewal with the hospital as I was unsure that I could keep the business going. Kylie was doing a great job managing OM1 and OM2 programs. However, even with her business skills, finances were tight.

Was this the end? No! The rollercoaster continued, and more big changes were hurtling my way.

# 7.

# My Heyday with OM

OMT was booming as we entered 2011. Kylie was at the helm of the business, and her talent, determination and energy were inspiring. She started the year with a teachers' retreat in Canberra to plan the many courses around Australia and the first course in New Zealand. Much of my time was spent recruiting and training teachers for our burgeoning business. I was regularly teaching in the Sydney hospital where the senior OM teacher was employed, but with no contract and tight finances, I had to think about options for running the hospital courses.

As more people became involved and shared my passion for this work, I knew that I had created something much bigger than me. There was joy and pride, certainly, and also an overwhelming feeling from the responsibility. Things happened so quickly – there was no time to pause, reflect or plan strategically. I lurched from one opportunity to the next and spent much of my time playing catch-up. It felt like one minute I had the idea to bring OM to Australia, and the next I was sitting in hospital board rooms trying to understand impenetrable legalese!

## Taking OM overseas for the first time

To keep the OMT teaching program going, we needed full courses to give our teachers work and ensure they stayed engaged with our organisation. They were all talented therapists who ran their own clinical practices and made a reliable income. My teaching role changed to teaching OM1 and OM2s around the country to fill gaps. We also took OM overseas for the first time. The senior teacher and I flew to Hong Kong to teach OM techniques to occupational therapists who had trained in Bowen therapy with ISBT. There were 42 students, all with English as a second language. The genuine hospitality of the students made the task doable – and we decided to never teach a group that large again.

We also taught OM1 and OM2 in Auckland, New Zealand. Whenever I needed to leave the room to negotiate access to tables or organise morning tea, the senior teacher taught on, further developing her excellent teaching style. This truly amazing woman rose to every challenge, and she just loved New Zealand.

## Decisions, decisions...

After so many years of cold calling, making contacts, talking the talk, persuading, cajoling and often feeling as though I was banging my head against a brick wall, it finally happened: someone called me! That 'someone' was the team developing the Olivia Newton-John Cancer Wellness and Research Centre (ONJCWRC) at the Austin Hospital in Melbourne. Later that month, I flew to Melbourne to meet Christine Scott, who was developing the blueprint for the wellness centre. My entire body smiles when I remember that first meeting, an informative chat that immediately established my trust in Christine and her vision for the ONJ facility.

Christine's crowded office overlooked the site earmarked for the development of a new high-rise building. This area would become the wellness centre, the new cancer treatment centre, research labs and, on the top floor, the palliative care ward.

There were piles of paperwork everywhere, and just enough room for us to sit knee to knee. News of my work at the Sydney hospital had preceded me and I glowed with pride as Christine reported what she had been told by her colleagues. We planned a series of meetings to begin nutting out the details.

As I flew home to Canberra that evening my head was awash with all the possibilities and the big decisions that lay ahead.

I knew that we couldn't afford to run the in-hospital program across two states, considering the costs for accommodation, travel and meals for two teachers for a week, venue hire and the limit of six fee-paying students per course. The fees couldn't increase as they were already among the highest for massage training in Australia. Hospital accommodation and meals were more affordable in Sydney than the Melbourne options, but in Sydney the teaching room hire kept going up without explanation. On some level, I felt like the Sydney hospital was giving me the opportunity with one hand and making it financially impossible with the other.

The hidden costs of in-hospital training, wherever it was taught, were alarming. Every student needed a police check and a working with vulnerable people card. Teaching and massaging in a hospital required a different insurance arrangement from the usual professional indemnity and public liability policy that massage therapists carry. Kylie put many unpaid hours into the paperwork for every teacher and student.

In Sydney, our well-respected senior teacher worked in the hospital where we taught, and she knew her way around and was aware of OM supporters and sceptics. However, the DON had not employed another OM therapist in over two years. I was acutely aware of that broken promise as it affected the therapist profoundly.

A plus for the ONJCWRC offer was that it was a three-year contract for two courses each year, with six therapists in each course. The Austin would pay for the ethics committee processes (although I still had to do a lot of work explaining course content to the ethics lawyers) and the hospital also let us use a 'mock ward' and a conference room for free. Christine talked about building a massage team and starting research as soon as our training was up and running. At the time I was a touch suspicious, because of the Sydney experience.

I decided to take a chance on The Austin. Christine Scott was a superb leader, inspiring confidence every step of the way. Her colleague, Tammy Boatman, was a compassionate and experienced occupational therapist. I asked them why they weren't setting up their own OM training program as there was a massage school across the road from the hospital. Christine replied that they didn't know enough about the massage industry in Australia and assessing the suitability of students was a highly skilled job. Wow! I felt valued and understood.

I met with the Sydney DON the following week to let her know of my decision to go to Melbourne. She was gracious and mentioned that the hospital had plans to develop their own massage training program. Apparently, their obstetricians were successfully bringing private massage therapists into the maternity wards. I offered any help I could give the massage program developer – and that was the last time I visited that hospital.

> This was a confronting moment when I realised that my hope for regulation of medical massage therapists was unlikely to happen. I am acutely aware of the gaps in massage training and the need for further training when therapists massage medically compromised people. If you know the doctor and he 'likes' you, therapists get to volunteer or be admitted as a contractor in a hospital, paid by private health insurance. How does the therapist get paid for travel time, or worse, waiting

time while the patient is taken to an X-ray? There is a huge amount of job satisfaction in this work, and the good heart of therapists is easily exploited. Don't get me started – my dad was a Labour man and family dinner conversations often involved lively political debate!

## Melbourne, here we come

Christine Scott and I kept in close contact through 2011 and I made a few visits to the hospital as the ethics committee processed the course content and I developed an understanding of the 'blueprint' Christine and Tammy had in mind. I told them what I had learnt over the past five years about OM and OM training in the US and UK. I shared the Society for Integrative Oncology (SIO) conference material and tapes, the S4OM lectures, contacts and research references, and my vision for respectful integration of OM into The Austin.

About halfway through the year, Christine used her Churchill Scholarship grant to visit the UK and US, including many of the places Gayle MacDonald and I had been to in Scotland, as well as the Bristol Clinic in England. In the US, she went to Memorial Sloan Kettering Cancer Centre, New York, and M.D. Anderson Clinic in Texas among others. It was an extensive tour and she worked very hard. The report she produced contained everything needed to establish an Integrative Medical (IM) service in Australia.

One of the OMT teachers, Kate Butler, joined me on this part of the 'OM at the Austin' ride and was pivotal to the successful integration of OM into ONJCWRC. Kate is highly educated, an excellent communicator, humble and confident. Every time I went to Melbourne, Kate picked me up and drove me around, any time of the day or night. Kate listened to my concerns, my joys and my worries. She provided wise counsel and great support.

> I remember one day we spent about four hours with the lawyer (a really lovely lady) working out a challenging bit of the contract (I think I was putting my home at risk if I got sued) and when Kate and I left the room and rounded a corner, we burst out laughing. When I drew breath, I asked Kate, 'Did you understand any of that conversation?' We laughed even harder. Legal language is an acquired skill.

## Bringing the oncologists on board

Through this busy year, we had worked out the ethics of teaching massage in the hospital, Austin Health had paid for all the legal costs and the ONJ team approved the uniform of green polo shirts emblazoned with 'Oncology Massage Therapist' in bright orange. Were we ready? There was one more task: deliver a technical lecture to all the oncologists. Easy!

> What memories I have of that day. The senior doctor (the boss) was my strongest supporter. All 32 doctors specialising in cancer management gathered for my talk. I was in my 'heyday' of public speaking, confident in my topic and passionate about my vision. Everything seemed to be going well. The PowerPoint was ready to go, the room filled up and just as I was about to start Christine whispered, 'Don't mention Ian Gawler or Petrea King.' Oh no! The first three slides were about how I taught myself OM at Petrea King's retreat centre. I started my talk like a fumbling, bumbling, nervy person. I improved as the medical facts emerged and at the end of my presentation the Boss stood up and said 'Oncology massage is coming to The Austin. If you have any questions now is the time to ask Eleanor, she is

> the expert.' There was a lot of politics in integrative medicine ten years ago. Maybe it is still the case?

Christine and Tammy made good use of my visits and I often turned up to a schedule of 'talks' to small groups of nurses, nurse unit managers (NUMs) and registrars. Kate and I had long conversations about how we could allay reservations about patient safety, and we spoke a lot about what we *wouldn't* do. We were not going to scrub, bruise or 'hurt' their patients in any way. If I couldn't convince someone in the meeting, Christine or Tammy put time into one-on-one meetings to sort things out. OM in a big, respected hospital was an experiment and we were all under the microscope.

The haematology oncologist meeting was memorable. People with blood cancers often have low platelets, bruise easily and deteriorate very quickly. Could OM therapists be trusted to massage haematology patients?

> Christine Scott took me to a small tearoom to meet the senior haematologist. He asked me to show him the pressure I would use to massage a patient with low platelets. I did my usual 'global release' technique for about a minute while he closed his eyes. He opened his eyes, looked me in the eye and said, 'Of course you can work with my patients.'

### The first courses at ONJCWRC

I developed information sheets and flyers and in January 2012, I flew to Melbourne to meet the ONJ team for the final time before bringing OM students to The Austin. We ran the first OM3 course at ONJCWRC in mid-March and the first OM4 in late April. The green shirts were a great success, the students were carefully selected and the 'mock ward' was easy to use. The senior teacher from the Sydney program and Kate taught the therapists and I rode 'shot gun', keeping my eyes peeled for any potential problems. Keeping Christine and Tammy up to date with progress was essential as they carried the responsibility for the professional integration of OM into the Austin Hospital.

OM3 was rolled out in the same way as it had been in Sydney: getting to know the hospital, moving around without getting in the way and as far as massaging cancer patients went, it was pretty easy. The students only massaged two outpatients on the last day and the folk being massaged were pretty healthy. With the support of the ONJCWRC team, OM3 went extremely well.

Infection control and manual handling sessions were a breeze in the 'mock ward'. We set a 'treasure hunt' for the students to find their way around relevant parts of the hospital (thanks to Gayle Macdonald for this great idea), and we gathered for lunch to hear about their adventures. What increased was the assessment of the students. We developed a series of tests, both theory and practical, and set homework each night so that all the learning steps were recorded. Kylie sorted out all this paperwork and recorded student results. I needed to prove we were complying with S4OM standards, and exceeding them if possible, as well as honouring ONJCWRC'S faith in us. I hoped that OM Australia could lead the world (there is that little 'face first' baby again!).

OM4 was a whole new adventure, and our approach was based on all we had learned working in the Sydney hospital, with lots of (literally!) hands-on work for the students. The first round of 'cold calling' is the hardest. We work in an industry where people book in to see us and from the first contact, we know they are seeking out our skills. The hardest part of cold calling is the rejection: 'Would you like a massage?' 'No, I don't like them.' Or the patient's family member might say, 'Dad doesn't like massage', while Dad himself looks on longingly, clearly yearning for non-medical touch. I remembered how Gayle set up her students. She asked the NUM which patients might benefit from a massage, then the student approached the patient and said, 'The nurse suggested that you might benefit from a massage this morning. What time would you like me to come back? The massage will take about 30 minutes.' We all filled our 'dance cards' quickly, with our nervous egos intact.

Once the courses were running smoothly, I offered two massages a day to any senior person who wanted to understand our work. Even the hospital CEO came one day to check me out. He was more interested in my laboratory experience than my massage skills, as his heart was in research, and he had regular massages from his own therapist. I was delighted he came; in fact, I was extremely pleased that a small group of senior people came for a massage with me to ensure the safety of their patients. The reality is that some may never really approve of massage in a hospital setting and others will.

We took our students into every cancer area of the hospital except palliative care, as that ward didn't open to us until we had proved ourselves. We spread out around the hospital; two students and a teacher went into the radiation waiting room, day oncology chemotherapy infusion suite, post-surgery cancer wards and acute care, even barrier nursing areas where we donned full PPE. At that time our students were working in the 'old' hospital and even in the 'very old area', The Repatriation Hospital, a mile or two up the road from where the ONJ centre was being built. I thought it a good thing to work in the clean and efficient older hospital as most of the students would be working in outdated wards if they were lucky enough to get a job in their local hospital.

By week's end, every student had an experience of every treatment area. The week went very quickly, and students and teachers were all exhausted by Friday morning. At the last of many debriefing sessions, we sent the newly qualified OM therapists home with our contact details so we could mentor them through the days ahead. Sadly, nobody got a paid job in a hospital; most returned to their patch and worked successfully in the community or in their local hospital as volunteers. While their skills were valued by nurses at the 'coal face', most accounts departments thought that a 20-cent morphine patch was better value.

## The grand opening

On 2 July 2012, the ONJCWRC opened its doors. I was absolutely thrilled to be invited to demonstrate massage at the grand opening of the fully restored heritage building and the new multistorey facility.

The day started very early with Olivia Newton-John doing a live interview for a TV breakfast show from the foyer of the Wellness Centre. I was standing around wondering how it all worked when the technician asked if I wanted a set of earphones to hear the interview. As I put the earphones on, I could hear a countdown of 'three, two, one…' (just like in the movies) and Olivia spoke with the host. After the interview, Olivia asked us all a little about ourselves then went to greet the first 100 people to be ushered in. My job was to massage an employee's father, who was face down on the massage table. As the first 100 people moved through the facility, so too did the photographers from various news outlets. Olivia came to chat with me in the massage room, accompanied by the then Premier of Victoria, Edward (Ted) Baillieu.

My Heyday with OM

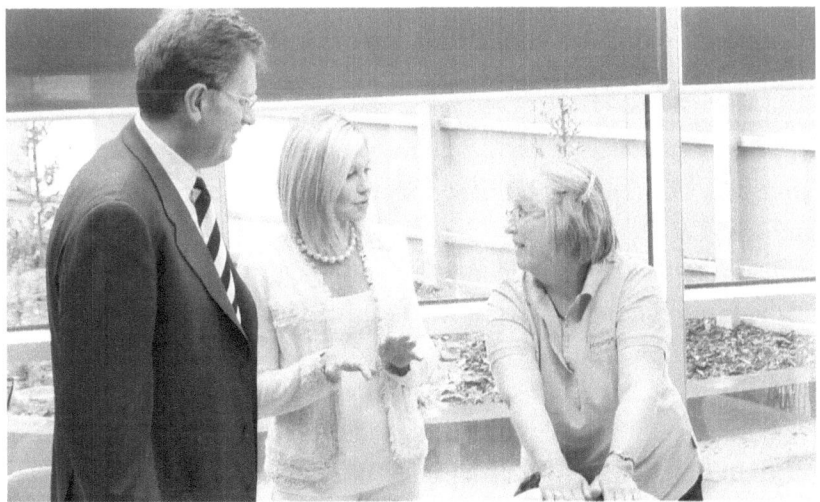

Olivia Newton-John included us all in the excitement of the day.

After the crowd moved through the Wellness Centre, they gathered in a small conference room where Olivia spoke to them. She told her story of cancer recovery and asked the audience to talk to her. It was all so heart-warming and inclusive. Everyone that had donated to the ONJ Centre came through the facility and had a chat with Olivia. Olivia took a short break between groups and then she just kept coming out to chat... all day long! It was fun to be part of this special day and my respect for her grew with each passing hour.

During one of the breaks, Olivia and I sat together. We established that we are the same age and still working hard, caring about our children and passionate about healthy cancer survivorship. Good lives well lived. I hope that the massage therapists in the ONJCWRC always maintain the highest standards and honour Olivia's vision and mine.

At 17, I learned to work in a hospital and, at 64, I was back again. I had worked in several different hospitals over my career and not a lot had changed. I felt so comfortable, even cheeky...

The in-hospital teaching team went back in late October and early November to run our second OM3 and OM4 programs in Melbourne. I had successfully moved the in-hospital training from Sydney to Melbourne.

The senior OM therapist from Sydney became the lead teacher of OM3 and OM4 at the ONJCWRC. During her service at the hospital, she had maintained her private practice and, on leaving the hospital, she walked into the open arms of her faithful clients. She committed to travelling to Melbourne twice a year to teach OM3 and OM4. This was totally necessary as students needed to see and hear her, learn from her depth of experience and understand that hospital work is different from any other massage job. As the co-facilitator of the OMT program, and later as the leader of the new ONJCWRC massage team, Kate, quickly gained experience and insights.

## Moving right along

There was no time to rest on our laurels after this excitement. Soon after the opening of the Wellness Centre, Kate started setting up the massage program with a firm promise from the powers that be that more OM therapists would be employed – and this time they were. By 2013, there were two other OMT-trained therapists employed part-time. Together with Kate, they worked in the Wellness Centre, on the wards and in the day oncology treatment areas.

Even with The Austin's focus on patient wellness, it was no mean feat to integrate complementary health services into a busy hospital. Kate was under considerable pressure to make it work, practically and financially. She recollects:

We knew the service would be popular, and that the pressure was on to prove its sustainability. I had to calculate precisely how much linen we required per week, how much oil we would use over what time period, and what equipment I needed, particularly for outpatients in the Wellness Centre.

When my supervisors and I talked about how many pre-booked sessions we could squeeze into the schedule, I knew from experience that the intensity of this work, while less physically demanding than remedial practice, can be systemically draining. I knew that there was a high risk of burnout. I also knew that by the time a patient arrives for a pre-booked appointment, I've confirmed their medical history, established how they are currently feeling, made an agreement with them as to what they might like or can expect from the massage and made them comfortable on the table (which can take quite some time when padding around medical devices, surgical sites and other complications). I need to establish their trust by taking it slowly, but then, when they are rousable from a more relaxed state and dressed, I need to check them off the system and record my notes in the hospital electronic records, change the full set of linen and reset the table. With so many elements to every single session, it became clear that anything less than an hour would not be enough time to deliver the quality of work that makes oncology massage so powerfully effective.

All eyes were on us in every situation. Kate's story about her first day in the chemo suite highlights the intensity we worked under:

> I became aware of some tense talk between two of the nurses nearby. It seemed to be about me, but I didn't know why. I figured that my work was very new to them, so I kept going, trying to focus on the task at hand, creating a bubble of peace and calm between myself and the patient in the midst of all the bright lights, the loud conversations, the bleeping chemotherapy pumps, the visiting specialists, volunteers offering drinks, dieticians, occupational therapists, family members and intermittent announcements over the hospital PA that there's a code blue somewhere within this small city that is The Austin.
>
> On completion, I went to wash my hands. A nurse approached me and asked, 'Why did you use purple gloves?' I had forgotten that purple gloves are exclusively used for handling cytotoxic drugs, and I had used them in the wrong context. In those early days, I was under constant scrutiny and seemingly small incidents such as these carried enormous importance.

Thanks to Kate's hard work, persistence in the face of opposition and her lovely way with people, the program flourished and many sceptics were converted into loyal OM supporters. In the end, the patients at The Austin were the winners, as countless anecdotes confirm. Kate continued:

> When you mention the word massage, most people think of kneading and pummelling, the 'no pain, no gain' philosophy. That's the culture we have created, and it requires constant explanation to educate both patients and staff that this is gentle touch, touch that is appropriate for people in vulnerable situations, and that this form of gentle touch can be extremely

> powerful if delivered skilfully and mindfully. After receiving a massage in the Wellness Centre, a patient said to me, 'That was gentle, and that was profound. I don't understand how something so gentle can feel so profound.'

One last beautiful story of Kate's illustrates perfectly the potential of OM and integrative medicine to benefit patient care.

> In the early days, an urgent request came through from the head oncologist for a patient to receive massage. She was extremely anxious, almost hysterical, at the thought of having a CT scan. It was an emotional cocktail of anticipating the claustrophobia associated with entering the CT machine – anxiety about what the scan would reveal and, in between sobs, a heap of issues relating to family abuse, current crises and financial challenges. She had needed scans before, and usually an anaesthetist was called to sedate her. On this occasion the anaesthetist was unavailable.
>
> I asked her to take a deep breath, remove her shoes and get onto the table in the position in which she would sleep. She curled up in a foetal position. I covered her with a blanket and for the next 35 minutes, stroked her back in a slow, deliberate, predictable, repetitive pattern. Her sobbing subsided and her breathing slowed down. She dozed in a half-waking, half-sleeping state. She was exhausted. I left her asleep in the care of a hospital volunteer. I heard later that her CT scan was performed without issue.
>
> I wondered about the comparative cost to the hospital of a nurse, an anaesthetist, and the drugs needed to calm her, compared to

40 minutes of my time. I also questioned the cost to her already compromised liver of having to process the anaesthetic drugs, compared to the bliss hormones (anandamide) that the massage was releasing into every cell of her body.

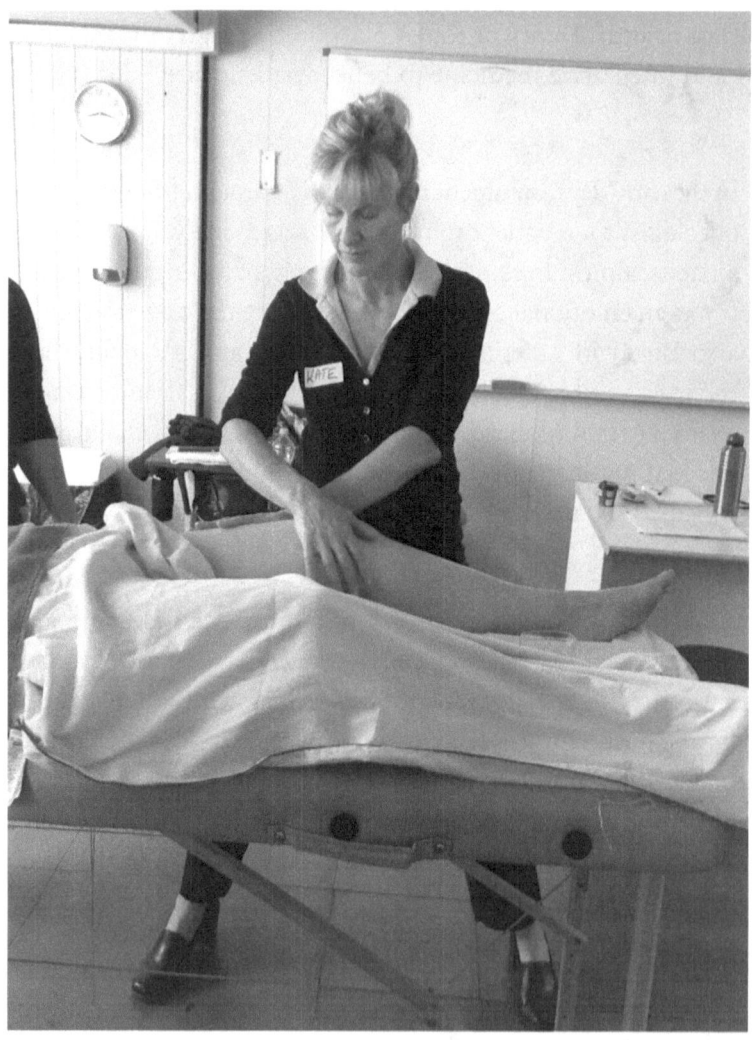

Kate in her OM cocoon demonstrating the leg sequence.

## But that's not all

Having a team of skilled, passionate colleagues meant that I had time to explore other opportunities to enrich OM and expand its horizons.

### An international visitor

Jamie Elswick, a scar management expert from the US, visited Australia in the middle of the work at ONJCWRC. I met Jamie at the S4OM conference in 2009 and asked her to come to Australia to teach us her techniques. Kylie sorted the finances and OMT flew Jamie from Anchorage, Alaska, to Adelaide, South Australia – about as far apart on the globe as it gets!

In Adelaide, Chris and I gave Jamie a couple of days to rest then we took her to Kangaroo Island for a day (her request), back to Adelaide and some sightseeing, up to the Barossa Valley then over to Daylesford in Victoria by car.

In Melbourne, Jamie ran a workshop for over 20 therapists. The Breast Cancer Network of Australia (BCNA) was the main advertiser, however I was surprised when on day one of the course, the CEO of BCNA wanted to immediately put the names of all the participating therapists on their website. I respectfully declined as I needed to check the therapists out myself. Not all the attending therapists had done OM1 and OM2 and I had to protect my 'brand', as well as folk with cancer.

After the stint in Melbourne, Jamie taught in Sydney and then the Sunshine Coast in Queensland. We flew our Perth teacher to Brisbane and OMT financially supported all OM teachers to attend the course. It was a wonderful time until Jamie declared on the last day that we couldn't write any of her techniques into our manuals, even if we acknowledged her work. Jamie had copyright and we respected that request. Jamie's tour was very successful and all the therapists attending her course eventually were listed on the BCNA website.

### Palliative care

The senior teacher and I ran the first palliative care course for OM therapists in Clare Holland House (a hospice) in Canberra in November 2012. Over the previous ten years the work of Wilma, a dedicated massage therapist, created and sustained a palliative care massage service in Clare Holland House, funded by Palliative Care ACT through donations. The nursing team at the hospice respected the massage therapists and were keen to teach day one of the weekend course. The nurses taught us about how the hospice functioned, general patient care and how the massage service fitted in. OMT taught day two: massage techniques, signs of dying and how to manage them, who to ask for advice or assistance in the medical team, and, very importantly, what to say or not say when working with an 'end of life' patient. We had a lot to share with our students after more than two years of in-hospital massage experience. It is challenging to create a 'bubble' of stillness while working in a hospital, as Kate described. However, in the corridors of Clare Holland House, there was an abiding sense of peace and gentleness. Unfortunately, and despite our best efforts, the palliative care course was not financially viable due to restrictions on student numbers, and after running it for a year, we had to stop.

### Another mountain to climb

To top off this tremendous year, I was invited to join the advisory team at the Chris O'Brien Lifehouse at Royal Prince Alfred Hospital (RPAH), Sydney. The first meeting was in an executive board room overlooking the Sydney Opera House, the Harbour Bridge and Circular Quay. I met a group of about 20 folk from a variety of professions, mostly medical and financial. I sat and chatted with the Dean of Medicine at Sydney University. All the CM people (foot reflexologist, yoga and meditation practitioner, aromatherapist and me) were asked to prepare a presentation about their speciality and present it at subsequent gatherings. I went first. At the next meeting, I arrived a bit early, so I set up my trusty PowerPoint slides (the ones that went down well at The Austin oncologists' meeting) and waited. I gave my talk to the other three CM professionals and two bankers. There was not a single medical person in the room. I imagined it was only OM that frightened them, but no, over the next few weeks, each CM person spoke to a group that was getting smaller and smaller! A heart-stopping disappointment, hot on the heels of our wonderful experience at The Austin.

The massage service that eventually developed at the Chris O'Brien Lifehouse has been running for over seven years. Two OML teachers who took part in the first in-hospital training program set up the OM service and one of them works there still, gradually making inroads into in-ward therapeutic acceptance. I advised the team about equipment, but Lizzie Milligan and Tania Griffin did all the work.

The Chris O'Brien Lifehouse is a world-famous centre of medical excellence that includes CM services. Looking back, I am overjoyed by the magic of OM being included at the birth of the centre, yet heavy hearted because I believe that the project didn't meet the vision that Chris and Gail O'Brien imagined as they scooted around Sydney seeking CM for Chris as his life drew to a close. I have read Gail's book and I remember her in the meetings of the advisory team. She was inspiring and clear about the role the centre would play in the treatment and survivorship of folk with cancer. I hope one day there will be an in-ward massage team who are salaried and supported by the medical professionals at RPAH. Maybe even an OM teaching team attracting massage therapists from around the country who take compassionate touch back to rural Australia. Now *that* would be something!

# 8.

# Time to Move On

So much had happened in such a short space of time. In 12 years, I had become the go-to person for all things oncology massage in Australia. I had been nominated twice for the Australian of the Year Awards (2009 and 2011) and the Telstra Small Business Award (2003) as well as establishing OM training in two major cancer hospitals. A highly skilled team of OM teachers was running courses around Australia and New Zealand. Kylie and the OM Board (which I was on) were running the organisation efficiently and it seemed like the sky was the limit!

In 2013, I continued to teach OM1 and OM2 when needed as well as riding 'shot gun' for OM3 and OM4 in Melbourne and palliative care courses in Canberra. I was involved in mentoring and teacher training all year round, as well as presenting at conferences. Everything seemed to be going well. Courses were filling up and our teachers were earning a good income from OMT.

However, some cracks were beginning to show. I was poorly resourced and lacked the skills and training to carry the responsibility for this rapidly growing organisation. I had worked so hard, for so long, all on a shoestring. I was exhausted. Money around OM was always tight and still is. Chris was now a Commander in the Royal Australian Navy and he had done extensive management courses over the years to create a skill set that matched the job he was doing. I could clearly see the differences in our skills and still, I foolishly rejected his offers to help me manage the business.

I have a competitive spirit and a stubborn streak. Something had to change, and it was me.

### OMT grows up

When OMT became OML in 2013, things became more serious and management and governance processes were tightened up. The Board decided to pay for a business consultant for Kylie and she found a person she could work with in Brisbane. This started a chain of events that changed everything.

Kylie's business advisor thought that she needed to run OML from Canberra and she wanted to be closer to her much-loved father, who was still recovering after a heart attack. Tubi, with her daughters, decided to move back to Canberra from South Australia, and together we rented a house in a leafy suburb with an excellent primary school. A year's lease gave us time to sell the farm and gave Tubi the time she needed to find her feet as a single mum. Sharing a home with our daughter and wonderful grandchildren somehow gave me space and time to notice what was happening to my place in OML.

> I have always wondered what it would feel like to retire. My dad was forced to retire at 65 (this was business policy in the 1970s), and he lived until he was almost 92. For almost 30 years, his skills and experience were not valued. My dad was an

aircraft engineer, acting as Production Foreman of Prestwick Airport from 1940 to 1952. He 'kept the planes flying' during WWII and emigrated to Australia to build a life of education and prosperity for his family. In his retirement, my mum kept him busy fixing neighbours' lawn mowers, fly screens, cars, and later, TVs. It was only in his inner circle that he was respected and his opinion sought. The world looked at him as old and past his 'use by date'. He knew everything, even when I was a grown up. Would ageism do the same to me in the enlightened 21$^{st}$ century?

I began to feel increasingly sidelined, even though I was still the 'face' of OM in Australia. There was a sense that the business needed to operate on a more professional footing than I had ever managed. I was part of the old 'fly by the seat of our pants' ways, where OMT lurched from one opportunity to the next. Things were changing and I didn't know what was happening anymore. I didn't seem to know what questions I needed to ask. I remember that we drove to Sydney to speak to a big, well-established massage training organisation with the view to selling OM training. I felt like I was the minor player, with no one interested in anything I thought or said. I felt achingly sad on the long drive home.

It turns out that mixing family and working relationships can be fraught! It worked incredibly well for a long time but, as the business became more successful and the stakes got higher, so did the potential for old family patterns to emerge, and it became increasingly difficult for Kylie and me.

At the time, it felt like everyone was seeing me as the problem. The business manager said to me, 'If I had to work with my dad, I'd *kill* him.' I met with a board member to discuss my concerns and he said, 'Think about what it's like for Kylie working with her mum.' The third person I sought advice from, a business development coach with whom Kylie and I had worked, referred to my age (65) three times in a single paragraph of an email.

I felt cornered and had a growing sense of irrelevance and injustice. What was I to do? Bow out gracefully and lose my life's work? Throw myself back into it? I decided to let go (a bit) by taking a sabbatical in Europe to think things through.

During all the business turmoil our farm sold, and Chris and I decided to build a new house that was closer to 'town' and still close to our farming community. The builder we chose was a dear friend, so we told him what we wanted, and in April 2014, we flew to Italy.

## Flying away

We had been to Italy briefly in 1972 on a Cosmos Tour, rushing through seven countries in 16 days! In our early 20s we were young and silly, and we loved the light-hearted feel of Italy. In 2014, friends recommended a B&B run by Aussie expats in a wee village called Polinago, south of Modena. Mt Cimone filled the horizon and the rolling hills between created the perfect adventure playground for keen walkers like us. Polinago will stay in our hearts forever. We were the only visitors in the village and didn't leave for three weeks. Everyone knew us and our coffee awaited as we walked through the café door. Our B&B retreat provided the perfect healing place for my mind and body. Our hosts trusted us to care for their pets while they took a break and we relaxed into the slow, welcoming pace of Polinago.

# Time to Move On

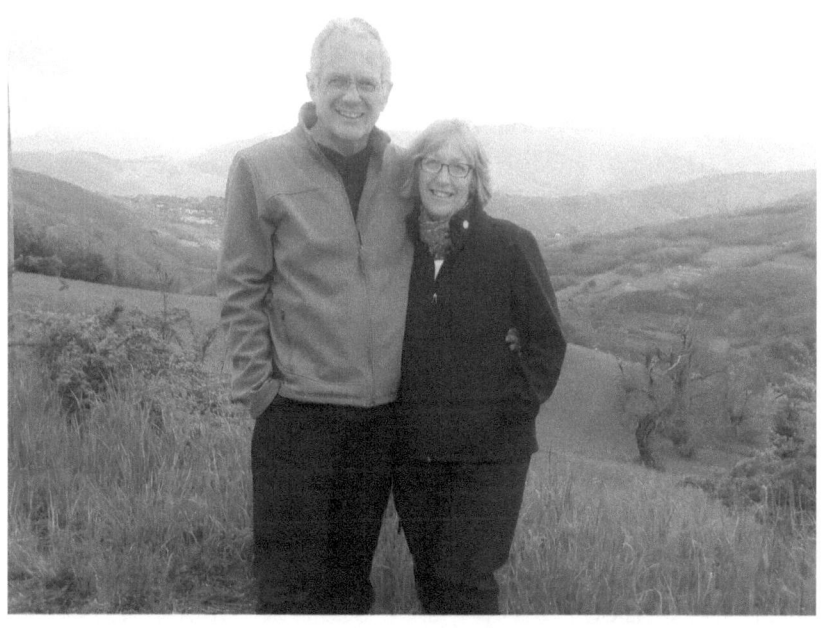

Rambling in the foothills of Mt Cimoni with
the love of my life – a healing time.

Our friend, Colleen, came to stay for a few days as part of an extensive European holiday and agreed to join us for some walking in Scotland. After five weeks in Italy, we flew to Scotland and settled into Skilmorely, at the mouth of the Clyde River. We spent six weeks there, lunching at the Gypsy Cream cafe, travelling to whisky-making islands like Dura and Islay and walking the West Highland Way – 100 miles from Glasgow to Fort William.

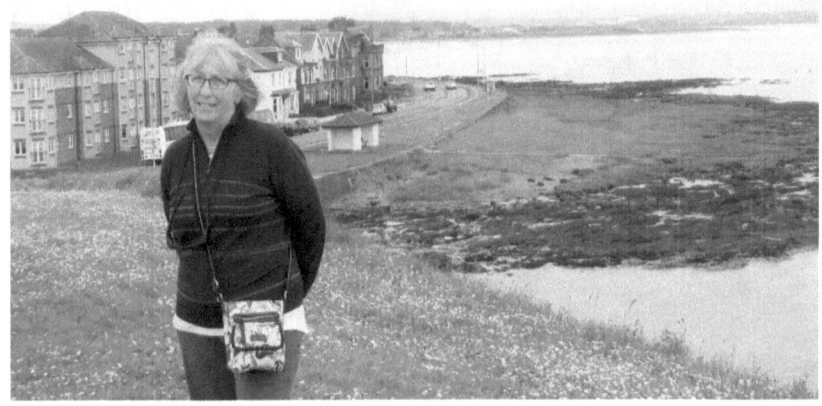

Troon, the seaside town in Ayrshire, Scotland, where I was born.

I felt a deep connection to my roots while walking in the Scottish wilderness. It was beautiful, wild and windy and it rained most days. One evening, I walked into a rack designed for our boots to dry overnight. My little toe swelled and instantly turned bright blue. I strapped my foot into the stiff, dry leather shell of my boot the following morning (ouch) but only managed another 50 metres before turning back to the hotel. The desk clerk arranged for a delivery truck to take me to the nearest jetty, where I could catch a boat that linked up with local buses to take me to the next hotel on our trek. I crossed Loch Lomond, the only passenger on a small ferry. In mist, on still water I sat with my thoughts. 'If nothing wrong is happening, what do I have to learn from this?' I asked myself.

Colleen and Chris were tramping through heavy rain on mountainous slippery slopes – a parallel adventure – and I felt very alone, stopped in my tracks by my crippled foot. After the solitary boat trip, I hobbled through the little village to find a local bus heading north. I entered a stately old guesthouse to ask directions. To my horror, the welcoming smile of the young receptionist opened the floodgates to my tears. I was in so much pain, so alone, yet being in a foreign land never crossed my mind. I boarded the bus after a medicinal cup of tea in the guesthouse and struggled to my destination. I sat in the bar with my leg propped up until the sodden walkers arrived. The bartender brought me terrible coffee and stale oatcakes that nevertheless tasted delicious.

Throughout that painful, lonely day I felt at home – the home of my father's father. Was this epigenetics at work? Maybe…

## Drawn back into the world of OM

Gayle MacDonald stayed with us in Skilmorely and we travelled to her clan's homeland. She had been to Scotland several times before, but never to visit the earth of her forefathers. We had great fun and it was touching to see Gayle connecting with her ancestry.

Gayle also took me to the Maggie Centres in Glasgow. These are facilities across the UK that offer free support to anyone with cancer and their families. I enjoyed every minute of our personal tour. The centres were beautifully fitted out and decorated, friendly staff offered us a 'cuppa' and the patients were welcoming too. In an area where medical staff were banned, patients had the privacy to speak their mind without fear of hurting feelings or being influenced by responses from doctors and nurses. We were told that this area was very popular and filled a therapeutic need.

Right next door was the local hospital that offered OM, counselling and a 'cuppa' in a Wellness Centre on the top floor, adjacent to the day infusion unit. All the chemotherapy chairs looked out over expansive views of Glasgow and beyond to Ben Lomond. Gayle and I spoke with the staff, and with their help, we explored ideas that might influence our own communities.

Gayle invited me to attend a one-day mini-summit in Nijkerk, The Netherlands, at which I met OM leaders from Ireland, Scotland, Amsterdam and Belgium, as well as 50-plus therapists. Gayle presented an afternoon workshop on how to ensure your client is completely comfortable before you begin an oncology massage. It was fascinating. The essential role of the medically proven relaxation response was again in the spotlight, a reminder of the need to empower clients with a sense of control when their lives feel totally out of their hands.

It was a wonderful day and for the first time I sat on an expert panel for a Q&A segment. I felt honoured and humbled, and I realised how much I had learned and could share about developing OM training to the highest standard. I believe that if we stand together as the new paradigm develops, strong in our basic skills and theory, we will open a respectful door into integrative CM.

In July, we left Scotland and went sailing on a small yacht around the Croatian coast, then popped back to Polinago for a festival, retraced our steps to Scotland to tour with Tubi and our granddaughters and returned home in September via a 60$^{th}$ birthday party in Malta. What a wonderful experience that was. The party was on the roof of a luxury hotel overlooking Valetta, beside a sparkling infinity pool. That movie star feeling washes over me again as I remember it all.

For five months, I had put all my feelings and emotions around OML in a velvet bag with the drawstring pulled tight and left it on the aircraft out of Sydney. Living in the present moment every minute of every day was therapeutic. While flying home, I scanned my physical body, and I knew that I had changed. Mind and body were relaxed, balanced and alive with optimism. I felt ready to come home and 'roll with the punches', as my mum always said when she felt powerlessness threaten to swallow her up. I was ready to wait for doors to open where my skills and experience were wanted.

## Home again, home again

We moved into our new house just before Christmas 2014. By late January 2015, we were settled, and I started working three days a week in a local multidisciplinary CM clinic. I attended Board meetings for OML. Having been away for so long helped me to become reconciled with my new situation. I was happy to be involved in grant proposals and explore research possibilities, and I began talking to the Board about the opportunity to teach overseas. On reflection, I was trying to carve out a new role for myself. The teaching and teacher training were all being done by capable experienced folk, the business was staying afloat and the Board was changing.

I was not ready to retire, as my heart still burned with passion for OM.

My diary for 2015 shows a mixture of trips and work. We walked the Larapinta track west of Alice Springs, went to the north coast of NSW with friends, had a camping holiday in Tasmania that included a week on King Island with friends… oh, the cheeses and the pristine natural environment! I spoke at a conference in Tassie in September, and I kept working on grant proposals for OML.

## Australian research into OM

It all started with discussions with Western Sydney University (WSU) about a scoping study by the Iris Foundation that came out of Gayle's work in Scotland.

The Iris Foundation conducted a survey of cancer communities across Scotland, suburban to remote, and found that there was a high demand for oncology massage. The response was so strong that the Foundation decided to pay for all OM training done by Gayle MacDonald in Scotland. There are many similarities between the two countries. Both have large areas of wilderness compared to land mass, densely populated coastal regions and a similar proportion of the population diagnosed with cancer each year (around 39 per cent).

Professor Caroline Smith at Western Sydney University listened respectfully to the information about the Scottish oncology massage scoping study, and we arranged to meet again a few weeks after Christmas 2015. At our next meeting, in late January 2016, Prof Smith brought along three RNs who managed aged care facilities close to the university.

> All three women were interested in my work and a lively discussion developed around a research project based on dementia patients receiving a light arm massage, without oil, administered by volunteers. Anecdotally, nurses and carers have observed that light touch can settle frightened or frustrated dementia patients. I stayed calm but felt a growing anger within me. Would these nursing professionals put a partially trained nurse into an ICU? It takes training to ensure that a massage therapist understands all the problems that can affect arms! Primary or secondary lymphedema, skin lesions and muscle wasting, to name just a few. Medical massage is a skill that should only be taught to an experienced massage therapist. Therapists need to know what a healthy body feels like first before they work with the elderly or the frail. Thankfully, nothing came of the aged care research at that time – and it still needs to happen.

Despite this inauspicious start, a research project developed, and I was graciously included on the team. OML raised $10,000 through crowd funding to donate to the research project and of course the cost was much greater. The study involved a survey of cancer services in Australia, as well as a range of focus groups with people from diverse ethnic backgrounds and a variety of cancer diagnoses. An astounding 93.2 per cent of cancer services completed the questionnaire. A major finding was that 72 per cent of participants wanted massage, referred by their oncologist, as their preferred CM. It is a truly excellent research paper that clearly shows that integrative oncology (IO) is both wanted and needed in Australia.[18]

The conclusion from the abstract says it all:

> *IO is increasingly being provided in Australia, although service provision remains limited or non-existent in many areas. Mismatches appear to exist between low IO service provision, CM evidence, and high CM use by cancer patients. Greater strategic planning and policy guidance is indicated to ensure the appropriate provision of, and equitable access to, IO services for all Australian cancer survivors.*

I had great expectations for the possibilities resulting from the research paper but alas, nothing changed.

## My last role at OML

Things kept chugging along. As my position in OML changed, I was given a job statement which, in essence, was to be a figurehead.

---

[18] Smith et al (2018). *Integrative oncology and complementary medicine cancer services in Australia: findings from a national cross-sectional survey.* BMC Complementary and Alternative Medicine 18:289.

I had a respected reputation in the wider complementary medicine community from my public speaking and the OM development work with Austin Health. My relationship with Petrea King was influential, as we had built a mutually respectful friendship and shared many ideas and concerns.

The Board assigned me a second role to develop the overseas arm of OML, and while Chris and I were travelling in Europe, I had spent time in Spain making contacts and setting it up (more on this in Chapter 9).

OML had worked hard at establishing a team of high-quality teachers in Australia and New Zealand. Kylie ran a team-building retreat in Queensland in 2016 for 16 OML teachers from Perth, Melbourne, Sydney and Canberra, which proved to be a wonderful success.

In October 2016, OML held its most ambitious conference to date, with respected international speakers and skilled participants from around Australia and New Zealand. There were four therapists from Washington DC, who gave wonderful talks that were very helpful to the growing body of OM therapists in Australia. Each therapist followed their own path within the organisation and importantly, their passion and commitment were underpinned by a strong business structure.

William Collinge and his partner, Maggie Donahue, from Eugene, Oregon also gave a powerful workshop on the safe touch for carers program mentioned in Chapter 3. William and Maggie stayed with us and our strong friendship has endured to this day.

### When things fall apart

However, things began to fall apart despite our best intentions, and 2017 was a year of turmoil for me. I was expanding OM teaching overseas, as the Board had asked me to do, and a hot topic at OML was the protection of intellectual property. In July 2017, I taught my original course, MC&M, in the Netherlands and it worked well. I had a plan for OML to teach overseas and I was developing networks as new opportunities opened up. My problem was that I was feeling increasingly 'managed' and overruled and, after almost 20 years of pushing oncology massage 'uphill', I was burnt out.

In late 2017, I left OML, after the hardest three years of my life. Despite the success of the research, and the possibilities for teaching OM overseas, it became increasingly difficult for me to function within the organisation and on the Board. I felt I did not fit there anymore.

In the turmoil and heartache of leaving OML, I searched for why things had changed in my experience of OML. A wise friend referred me to a paper by Deane Juhan.[19] He describes six phases of development where organisations 'outgrow' their founders.

In phase one, 'A particular individual, with a particular talent and world view, is faced with a personal problem, or with a particular population of patients, and works out an innovative method of bringing relief and restored function.'

Briefly, I had an awakening that I developed into a training program. Others were also moving towards the awakening and found my course. Together, we refined the skills and became a teaching community. A new modality was born. Marketing began in earnest. A bureaucracy was born, and an institutional phase started.

In phase six, 'Things bubble along. The master ages and is less and less active, more withdrawn from the day-to-day teaching and operations. More and more responsibility – and authority – devolves to the board and office staff. Instructors and practitioners, according to their nature

---

[19] Juhan D (2005) Integration: Working In Bodywork's Big Tent: The Institutionalization of Human Potential. Available at: https://www.jobsbody.com/integration-working-in-bodyworks-big-tent-the-institutionalization-of-human-potential/

## TOUCHING CANCER

and their own human potentials, develop increasingly idiosyncratic ways of working and teaching.'

That was OML in a nutshell. Deane mentions several times in his paper that, 'There are almost never any villains,' and that none of the parties involved intend harm to others or to the organisation.

OMG has allowed me to hold onto the thread of my passion, recover my self-esteem and continue to live a purposeful life.

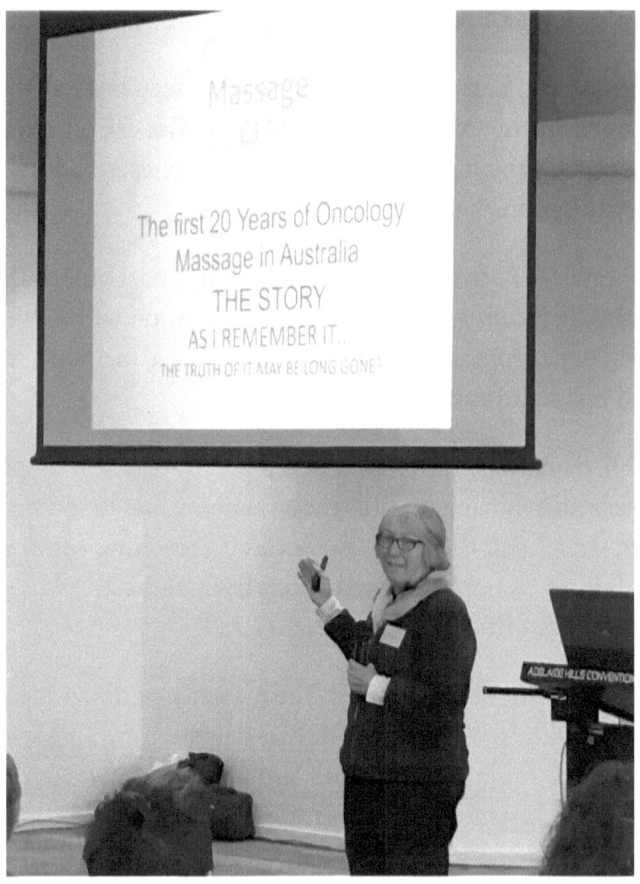

Presenting at the COSA conference at Darling Harbour 2017.

# 9.

# OMG Is Born

Once my place in OML was gone, I decided to build on the work I had recently undertaken in Spain. My family was a little worse for wear and I prayed that all the years of loving each other would eventually heal the wounds. I knew that OML was being run with the best intentions. I remained hopeful that we could work together in the future for the benefit of OM in Australia.

### The story of Spain

As with most things in my life, serendipity played a big part. The story started a while before I left OML, with Monica Moreno. I first met Monica in her clinic when I booked a massage, on the recommendation of a friend. Monica is a gentle soul with her own story of loss to cancer and she was drawn to OML training. One spring day, not long after we met, Monica told me that she wanted to take OM to Spain, and the seed was sown.

I really enjoyed the idea of taking OM to other countries. S4OM is excellent at promoting OM in America, however the complexities of regulation that vary from state to state made development of the OM industry difficult. Could our Australian course take the 'good news' to a wider world? Sounds a tad evangelical… I guess I've always been a crusader!

Within weeks of our first meeting, Monica and I became very comfortable in each other's company. After another conversation about the need for compassionate massage in Spain, as if by magic I opened my computer and booked two tickets to Barcelona. It was a very spontaneous decision!

All of our plans fell into place and in May 2016, we flew to Barcelona with Chris, my long-suffering benefactor. Before Monica and I began work in Madrid and Barcelona, Chris and I met Colleen, our walking partner, in Malaga, on the edge of the Mediterranean Sea. Colleen had just finished the 1000km Camino walk and we spent a week in the mountains around a White Village in the Sierra Nevada Mountain region of southern Spain as her 'walk-down'. It was warm, beautiful and felt magical.

Monica visited her family in the Barcelona region, and we met up again in Madrid. Monica took us by train to visit her uncle in Toledo. He met us in the old city and took us to his property just outside the city.

Their beautiful two-storey home emerged from a dry landscape which reminded us of Australia. Monica's aunt, a herbalist, had a kitchen table laden with drying herbs. We were offered a variety of teas that she brewed for our particular health challenges (I was exhausted again). In this family there is a strong belief in natural products, especially home-grown herbs and fresh vegetables.

Much of our time in Spain was made affordable through the generosity of Monica's family.

Another of Monica's aunts joined us on a visit to a Cava winery, in a town with champagne cork-shaped bollards lining the streets. On our short train trip from Barcelona to the wine district, Monica taught us some Spanish history. The return trip was a scary ride in a tiny car driven by her lively, generous aunt.

## Making connections

Now, our OM work in Spain awaited us. A doctor in New Zealand, who knew about my work at QFL and with OMT, recommended that we catch up with his friend, an intensive care specialist who was introducing compassionate interventions for patients in the ICU.

After a long train ride to the outer suburbs of Madrid, Monica and I walked to the hospital. I valued the trip as it opened my eyes to the hardships of outer city living, much as I had experienced in Western Sydney where I grew up. The road leaving the carpark at the train station morphed into a well-worn dirt track. We followed a stream of folk making their way on foot to the entrance of a large new hospital.

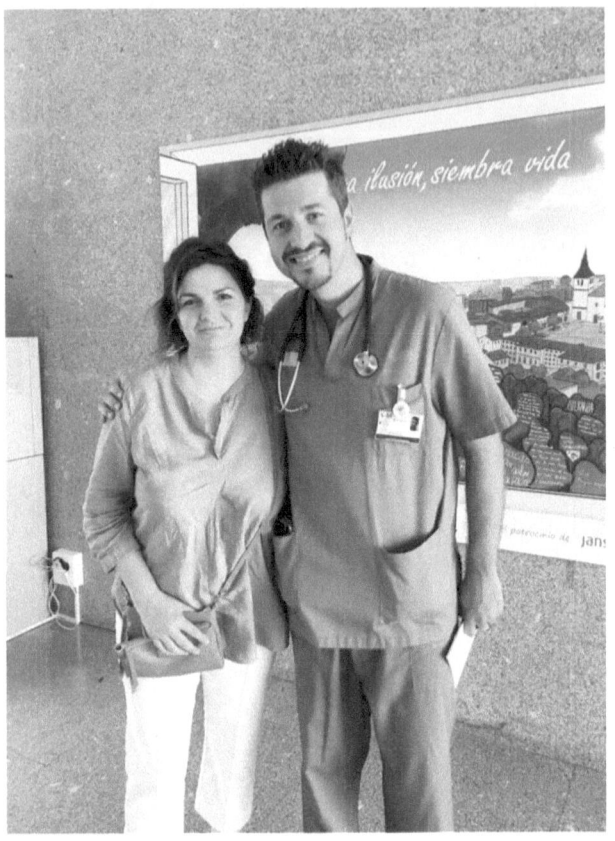

Monica and Dr Gabi Heras, Madrid 2018

Our host was expecting us. As we met, I felt a huge bundle of energy surrounding this young doctor and I was delighted that we had made the effort to meet him. He guided us to the 'rest-room' he used while on duty. Our conversation started, via Monica's skilled translation, on his vision and dream for ICU patients. We talked about the isolation of illness for patients and their families. The reality is that when folk are really ill, there is nothing to do but sit and wait for any improvement, or for death. The inspiration driving this young man was his ability to connect with his patients and he used that skill to connect with me, especially without a common language.

We talked about how his ideas might work, like a 'trip' from the ICU to a sunny spot outside, taking all the attached life support; then ways to bring music into the ward – not elevator music, music that was meaningful to the patient or their family – and how to convince staff to change, step outside their experience or imagining and let go of their fears.

If we always do what we have always done, we will always get what we always got. And what do we get? Sad, lonely patients and sad, lonely, powerless loved ones. We debated (via Monica) the role of safe compassionate touch like oncology massage and I learned about the high level of 'lotioning' that patients received in his ICU ward.

We were all on the same page. I was with a kindred spirit who was looking more tired as the minutes ticked past. I knew we needed to leave. A day's journey for a 30-minute chat in Spanish where I only understood half the content but smiling eye contact said it all. Many people have medical experiences just like this every day.

Before we said our goodbyes, I asked him if I could show him the pressure, speed and rhythm we used in an oncology massage, and he agreed. I positioned him on his day bed and began to massage his legs, then moved to his shoulders. By the time I got there, he was fast asleep, the best compliment for any OM therapist. Monica and I tiptoed out, made our way back to the main entrance and then onto a train bound for Madrid.

What had we achieved? We had no idea, so I looked out the window as Monica explained more of the scenery to me. Spain is beautiful, tough and much like any country with big cities, wealth and poverty sit right next to each other, day in and day out.

Chatting away, we were oblivious to the fact that we had pulled up in the main station for Madrid, where we had changed trains on our way out. I asked Monica if we should be getting off. Monica leaped up and headed for the electric doors which were soon to close. I followed but alas the doors closed in my face. There I was on a moving train to an unknown destination with Monica gesturing to me to catch a train back to her as soon as possible.

Between stations, I searched through my handbag. Surely, I had a phone number for Monica's uncle or the address of his apartment, where we were staying? No, I didn't. Nothing – not even my English-Spanish phrasebook. Smiling like a frightened puppy I disembarked and found my way to a train going back to Madrid Central. Where was Monica? I made my way to a series of ramps that allowed me to overlook all the platforms. Phew, there she was, looking as worried as I did. We hugged in relief, then caught a bus home to the sweetest part of suburban Madrid.

This was the neighbourhood where Monica lived as a young teenager, and I noticed how comfortable she was in her own skin. I feel privileged to have shared so many wonderful (and scary) experiences with her over the past seven years.

We were greeted with open arms at the little flat. Chris and Colleen had enjoyed getting lost and found again, tried Spanish tapas and generally exhausted themselves sightseeing in Madrid.

Research into the local massage community and cultural attitudes towards massage were constantly on my mind. I decided to seek out a local massage therapist and test the massage culture. The closest therapist was a university-qualified physiotherapist who was taught not to massage anyone with cancer or other major systemic illnesses. She gave me a lovely remedial massage and was very interested in my work. She acknowledged that the science I told her about made sense, then suggested that I speak with her professional association. We found the association office the next day in the city. Unfortunately, the front desk person was no help except for a phone number we could try when time allowed. Sadly, time never allowed. This is typical of my experience; there is never enough time or money to develop the opportunities that unfold when I talk to people about OM.

In Madrid, Monica took us to a café where we saw fantastic flamenco dancers, she guided us through beautiful shops, took us to the local swimming pool to do some laps and we all walked endlessly through famous parks graced by renowned art works. With Monica as travel guide and interpreter, we 'did' Madrid in style.

The train to Barcelona was busy and a little crowded. That might have been because I didn't book first class seats this time. Leaving Malaga without Monica, we were surprised to be given a meal with wine, like on a 'classy' plane flight. I had accidentally booked the most expensive seats. Monica had booked the trip to Barcelona which was considerably more affordable!

Colleen and Monica got on well. Colleen is a distinguished pastoralist, an experienced massage therapist and a traveller who is curious and interested in everything. We arrived in Barcelona and made our way to a B&B near the railway station. The next couple of days were not my best. The room was small and perched atop eight flights of stairs. That night I had my first ever panic attack due to claustrophobia and general exhaustion. We moved to a bigger hotel and everything improved.

Each morning, Monica and I made our way to find a massage school. With Monica's phone, we tracked them down, made appointments and 'cold called' like travelling salesmen. The first one we found was run by a lovely aging gentleman doctor who lived and worked in a splendid building in an expensive neighbourhood. I was thoroughly impressed by the marble stairs, an old internal 'birdcage' lift and antique furniture adorning the waiting room. Teaching massage and running a massage clinic including osteopathy treatments appeared to provide a good income!

Monica's humility and skill again charmed the host and he talked for some time with us. He fully agreed with our techniques, science and practical assessment program for the students. After considering the possibilities for developing OM training in Spain, he referred us to the Instituto Superior de Medicinas Tradicionales (ISMET). Debriefing in a nearby café after the meeting, we felt heard, valued and full of hope.

### First connection with ISMET

I think the director of ISMET knew we were coming, as we were quickly ushered into his very 'upstairs, back room' office. Monica took on her professional role and before long we were planning dates to return and teach. I was invited to speak at an international conference/expo in Barcelona the following year.

This was all too good to be true, as the old saying goes. The professional magic Monica brought to our meetings was delightful to watch and so much more than I imagined was possible.

It was time to share a final meal together in Barcelona, reminisce about all the sights we had seen, food we had shared and cultural awareness I was beginning to gain, all led by Monica's intimate knowledge of her much-loved homeland.

### Teaching in the Netherlands

Our little foursome split up the next day at the railway station. Chris and I went to holiday with friends in Paris for a week and then to The Netherlands where I taught OM at a massage school near our friend's home. Carla's first husband was part of The Netherlands' diplomatic staff in Canberra for five years. During that time Carla did oncology massage training with OML and I got to know her well.

I only had three-and-a-half days to teach massage therapists the basics of OM so I combined Modules 1 and 2 into a three-day program. The course came down to my original program called Massage Cancer and More (MC&M). It didn't rock the boat too much at OML, and still met the S4OM requirements.

Almost everyone spoke English, so Carla only had to interpret some of the more technical aspects of the course. It was good preparation for the development of the courses in Spanish that needed to be completely translated. Teaching in two languages is very time-consuming!

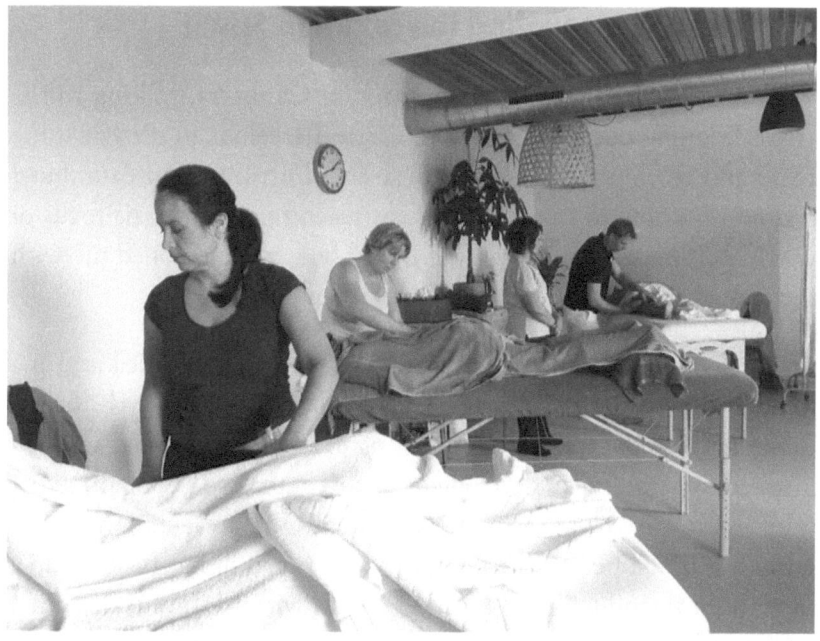

Carla observing the OM2 practical exam in The Netherlands.

The NUM from the local hospital was on the program and was very keen to establish a massage team in the cancer wards. The owner of the massage school was a published author of a textbook on the benefits of gentle massage, written in Dutch. There was the making of a resource for the NUM to develop. She had a steady stream of massage therapists coming through the local massage school, and the owner was keen to specialise in training hospital ready therapists. Yet again, there wasn't the time or money to develop the opportunity.

The class I taught was well attended, with eight qualified massage therapists ready to 'spread the word'. Many of them were already seeing clients with cancer and with Carla's clinic in a nearby town I felt optimistic that oncology massage would become a routine service in this area of The Netherlands. Through Gayle MacDonald, I also met OM teachers in Belgium and Amsterdam.

## Negotiating the return to Spain

Within a few short weeks, I was back in Canberra, talking to the OML Board about my desire to return to Barcelona to present at the Expo and teach an OM1 program. I could dream the dream, but I had no idea how to fund it. Overseas teaching was not the focus of OML's business even though the Board had commissioned me with the task of exploring Barcelona's interest in our program.

To their credit, the Board approved funds to fly Monica and me to Spain in April 2017. It was a tricky time for me at OML. In the time since I wrote the original training manuals, senior teachers had invested unpaid time in developing course content, so the Board didn't want me to 'give away' any course content. The presentation for the Expo was developed by the Board and they agreed that I could run a three-hour introduction to the OM course with Monica translating. I did rebel by teaching my style of leg massage and allowing it to be photographed. I was strongly attached to that technique, and I guess I 'got my knickers in a knot'.

Fifty therapists attended the introduction workshop. The workshop was exciting, and most attendees registered interest in joining the OM1 and OM2 classes when the teachers from Australia could come and teach. ISMET wanted to pin me down for a date, but I knew the tricky situation I was in at home. ISMET would have to wait.

OMG Is Born

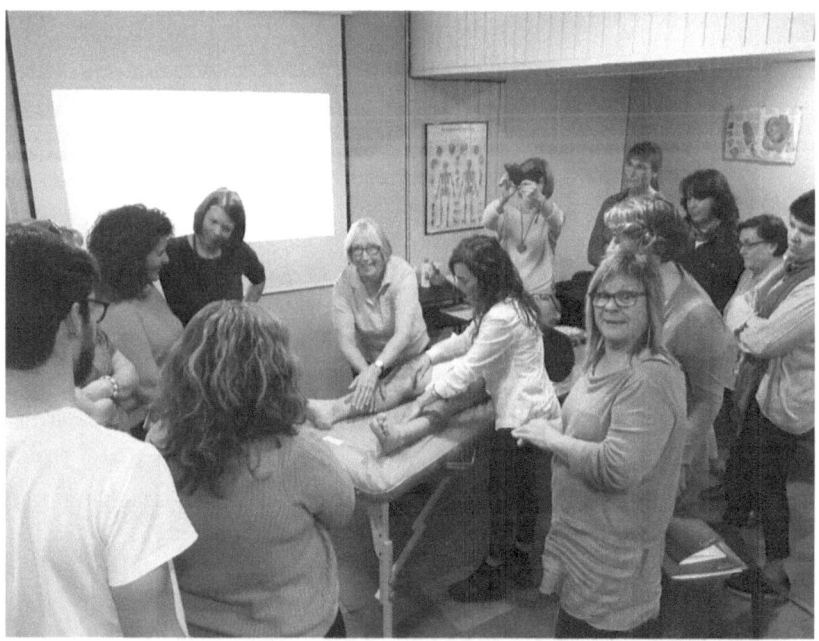

Introduction to OM in Barcelona, Spain 2017.

Over a hundred people attended my presentation at the Expo. By Australian standards, that was a lot of interested folk. In Barcelona, it was average for the 'breakout rooms'. A massive 23,000 people passed through the doors of the Expo in three days.

I had spent my own time and money developing a relationship with ISMET, I had visited the venue to ensure that the teachers and students were learning in a safe environment with a highly regarded CM training organisation, and I had developed a system with ISMET to record student results and suitability for further training or work in a medical practice. In 2017 I started discussing a teacher training program to provide ISMET with their own teachers over time.

By October 2017, ISMET had promoted OM and filled a class with 16 students. I knew that I was too tired to go back to Spain. Immediately Kate Butler (from ONJCWRC) came to mind. Kate was perfect for this work, and I knew her well.

Kate and Monica were preparing to teach OM1 twice in Barcelona. We needed two OM1 classes of 12 or more students to pay the bills. Just days before they left Australia for Barcelona, suitable accommodation was found for them and the second OM1 class filled up. Hooray. I imagined that God was 'winking' at us again.

Three potential Spanish teachers emerged from this first group in Spain. ISMET had handpicked the students so my faith in ISMET grew exponentially. Kate taught the program and Monica interpreted. Carla from The Netherlands came at her own expense to be a support person. They did a fantastic job. The feedback from students and management at ISMET was heart-warming. There were a few things to 'tweak' for next time, and OM teaching was up and running in Spain.

### Oncology Massage Global

Five months later, I was no longer involved with OML, I had purchased my intellectual property for the cost of my superannuation and I had established OMG.

With the help of my dear friend, Gracie, I set up my new business comprising two excellent teachers, Chris as benefactor (yet again), and the support of skilled friends in Barcelona. I had my own international business once again and OM was being taught in Spanish. Monica was a fast learner and she worked long and hard to establish a healthy relationship with ISMET.

As a free agent, OMG returned to Barcelona in March 2018 to teach an OM2 to complete the training of the therapists who did OM1 in October 2017. Kate and Monica taught two more OM1s and supervised teacher training in the last OM1. In a display of immense stamina and passion, they worked daily, except for two days, from 5 March to 23 March 2018. Thanks to ISMET, they were paid well.

Due to COVID-19, the last time OMG taught in Barcelona was in March 2018. Our colleagues at ISMET have been hit hard since 2019. I have stayed in contact with the CEO of ISMET and Monica has continued to support the partly trained teachers via text and phone. In early 2022, Monica and Kate are working with the Barcelona teachers so they can enrol as teachers with S4OM. ISMET has run a few OM1 programs, and they are waiting for OMG's return to run OM2 courses. Once the ISMET teachers pass the OM2 teacher training the new teachers can register with S4OM and they can teach OM1 and OM2 any time they have students.

Towards the end of 2019, a massage school owner, Marcelo, in Argentina contacted me with a story that really worried me. A therapist who had only completed OM1 with Kate and Monica in Barcelona was teaching OM in her own country. Marcelo's business partner took the course and noticed that all contraindications were absent. The enterprising therapist was in contact with doctors and massage teachers, and she presented at a medical conference in her own country without the precautions being spoken about.

So, what do I do? For 20 years I have been trying to 'massage' a respectful integration with the medical community and sharing only part of the course is not supporting my goals. I asked Marcelo to let this person know that I was happy to supply her with any research papers, PowerPoints and other teaching material that included the contraindications. I think my attitude caught my Argentinian friends off guard. OM training is not a competition, it's a team effort and it requires compassion at every level of the business.

In January 2020, I bought airfares for Monica and me to begin teaching in Buenos Aires. Thank you to Chris once again. However, due to COVID-19, the trip was unable to go ahead.

## Argentina and online

Monica and Kate developed an online version of OM1 in early 2021 and taught a group of 26 therapists (via Zoom) in Argentina. A group of this size was too big. Marcelo would not take my advice on this issue but he now runs classes with 14-16 students – still too big, as Gayle only takes eight students on her courses. It was divided into two groups for OM2, which went well.

Monica and Kate have been working hard at this project for over a year and have been recently assisted by Jodi Lawler who is a dear friend as well as an online teaching expert. Another 'wink' from God.

The OMG team all work for little or no monetary reward and we hope that, once the student platform is established, the business side of things will be much easier and money will flow (yep I'm still an optimist!).

Marcelo had recruited 14 students for OM1 in October 2021 – an oncologist, nurses, as well as massage professionals who had come from as far away as Mexico and Costa Rica. When the borders open again, there will be a demand for Kate and Monica to fly into Barcelona and Buenos Aires and demonstrate OM, fine-tune the teacher training and hand over to the local therapists. There is plenty of work for us all, so the adventure continues…

# 10.

# Then It Happened to Me

By 2019, I was in a much better place emotionally after a distressing few years. Time had healed some of the wounds, my family was coming back together, slowly but surely, and there were exciting prospects for travel and adventure with OMG.

Then everything changed. COVID-19 burst into our collective consciousness and upended our lives. However, a diagnosis of cancer in July 2020 that came out of left field affected me in ways I could never have predicted. I'm so human!

### More research in the pipeline

In late 2019, I began thinking about a new research proposal. OMG was going well, with Kate and Monica working hard on course content and translation, and I felt like I had another research project in me.

Through the Bowen Therapy Federation of Australia (BTFA), Prof Jon Adams from the University of Technology in Sydney called for expressions of interest in joining his research team. Jon has a unique interest in practitioner-based research, where therapists in a particular field contribute data from their practices and the collated data helps to improve the evidence base in the modality.

Bowen therapy is not accepted by the health funds for rebate status, despite the best efforts of the BTFA and the Bowen Association of Australia (BAA). Bowen practitioners remain in the 'doldrums', alongside other excellent complementary medicine modalities like yoga and naturopathy. What we all have in common is the lack of recognised, university-based research to prove our worth.

I didn't know Prof Adams well, but I liked his 'can do' approach to CM. I had seen him speak at the BTFA conference and in 2017, just as I was leaving the Board of OML, I invited him to tell the Board about his work. The OML 'contact-a-therapist' list had over 200 therapists trained through the same courses, which was perfect for Jon's style of research. On the back of the Western Sydney University research, I believed that the OM community would benefit from taking part in Prof Adams' practitioner-based research project, elevating OM nationally with some university clout. The OML Board were unable to invest in the project, which represented another missed opportunity due to a lack of funding.

The University of Technology in Sydney subsequently developed a practitioner-based research program at the Australian Research Centre in Complementary and Integrative Medicine (ARCCIM), called the ARCCIM International CIM Leadership Program. Three-year fellowships were conferred on practitioners elected to the international group and the plan was to meet in Italy in the European summer of 2020 to exchange ideas and insights into a diverse range of CM modalities. I applied for a fellowship spot.

With all of this exciting research unfolding, Chris and I booked a three-month holiday on the South Island of New Zealand, leaving on 3 March 2020.

Jon rang me in Christchurch on 12 March to interview me for the fellowship position, and later that month I received an email with an offer. It was a wonderful message, telling me how strong the field of international applicants were and how pleased they were to have me on their team.

I was overjoyed! I'm a team player at heart, and I had been walking a lonely road for quite some time.

## Then came COVID

The first week that Chris and I were in Christchurch, there was a lot of talk about COVID-19 in Australia, the panic buying of loo paper and so on. New Zealand seemed to have little to worry about and our B&B hosts encouraged us to stay on with them, mind their dog while they took a holiday in their caravan and guaranteed us a bed until we wanted to go home.

We went to a public lecture about COVID-19 at the University of Otago. It was interesting to hear such an honest assessment of the situation. The speakers told us that they didn't know what would happen and that we should be looking after older people and those who are shut-in, concentrating on provisions and ethical decision-making. There was a lot to learn about a global pandemic. When Qantas announced 'last flights' to Australia, we decided to come home and went into two weeks of isolation, emerging on April Fool's Day.

Meetings via Zoom with therapists in Argentina and Barcelona continued as the months went by amid growing, scary COVID news. Life for Chris and me was as good as it had ever been. We seemed to be happy, laughing a lot, and the tricky dynamic of having worked with my daughters in OML was slowly returning to a peaceful acceptance of family differences of opinion. As with transitioning through the teenage years, the 'bumps' hurt, but love gets us all through.

## A shot across my bow

Late one cold night in early July 2020, I developed pain in my left side that felt like a pulled muscle. The pain progressed around my torso towards my heart. Chris drove me to A&E and I was seen immediately. It wasn't my heart and the pain relief worked well. A very competent young female doctor asked me to have a CT scan. I was delighted to be given the choice! I could tell from the X-ray technician's demeanour that he had found something troubling. When the doctor arrived with a script in hand for high dose opioids, I wasn't surprised to hear that I had a compressed fracture of T12 (a thoracic vertebrae) and my blood tests were slightly abnormal.

Due to the COVID alert, I was sent home the next morning with an appointment booked to see a senior physician in a couple of days. Frustrated by having so little information, I asked my GP to go through the hospital records with me. He told me that multiple myeloma was a possibility and that I needed a series of tests to sort things out.

In a few short days, my world was turned upside down.

## Why me? Why now?

Cancer? Me? Why not me? 'You can never go back to the day before the diagnosis.' I heard my own words ringing in my ears.

For over 20 years, I have been challenging others to question the situation in which they found themselves and respond with curiosity, not fear. This is easy to say to other people and not easy to do yourself. This was a very hard lesson to learn.

I didn't label my state of mind 'shock' until weeks later when Petrea and Wendie came to visit and asked, 'Could you be in shock, do you think?' Of course, I was in shock. I'm an optimist by nature and I was taking aging in my stride. There was money in the bank, I could exercise easily, we ate well and our friendship group was supportive and generous. I was in great shape except for cancer. I couldn't, or didn't want to, believe the medical experts caring for me.

I have asked many clients at QFL, the massage therapists I have taught and clients in my clinic to think 'not why me but why now?' In my work, I have challenged people with my firm belief that what we think and feel changes the body. Often folk can pinpoint an event like the loss of a child, a divorce, or being caught in a disaster of some kind (flood, fire, storm, financial tragedy, etc) about 18-24 months prior to the diagnosis, when the epigenetic predisposition was activated because the fight or flight hormones went unchecked for too long. The immune system fell asleep.

What had I been thinking and feeling? I didn't know.

As discussed in Chapter 2, through epigenetics, cell surface receptors adapt all the time to our neurochemistry, the food we eat and the toxins that are unavoidable in daily living. Even though I knew the science, I took my cancer diagnosis very personally. Why me? I've been caring for and about people with cancer my whole adult life. Self-pity is so very comfortable and reassuring.

I know that what I eat matters. I have been eating SLOW (Seasonal, Local, Organic, Whole) food for decades. Our kids only had homemade pizza, and takeaway food was for holidays. I was the one with the reputation for making healthy cakes years before they were fashionable.

Many times, I have been told by people from all walks of life that food doesn't make any difference to our health. Food won't cure cancer (and food alone won't prevent cancer) but it does change our biology.

My retort is, 'What we eat today walks and talks tomorrow,' a quote from a billboard on the side of the railway line that I'd see on my way to work way back in 1967.

'Follow the food triangle, that's all you need to do.' 'Oh yes,' I'd say. 'The one that has been around for the last 40 years.' I have lived long enough to know that food fads, government-sponsored or not, are about making money. What is done to margarine to make it look like butter is another travesty of deceit…. and on and on I'd go.

So, what could I change? Not my food – I was adamant about that. I could fine-tune my diet and exercise, but more importantly, I needed to work on my 'self-talk'. What was I thinking and feeling and how was it affecting me?

At the time, I didn't have a clue how to find myself again. How long had it been since I sat quietly in meditation with a total focus on myself?

You know all the thoughts that slip into your head when you are 'thought-less' like, 'I'm fat; I must be greedy,' 'That dress looks silly,' 'I'm not good enough,' or worse things like 'mother guilt', focusing on my mistakes in life and the 'if only' trap. I had been totally unaware of these negative thoughts since leaving OML four years before. The separation felt like losing a child and I didn't allow myself to realise that until I was diagnosed with cancer.

My acupuncturist nailed it: I had 'taken my eye off the ball'.

Why a blood cancer? Why cancer in the haemopoietic pathways that are vital for life? Why couldn't I have a breast lump that could be cut out? The cancer cells in my body are the ones that make plasma, the vital fluid that carries the red and white blood cells around my body – I cannot live without them. They need to be poisoned with chemicals, the like of which I have been protecting myself from for half my life.

Why now, when life was feeling peaceful and happy?

## Onto the conveyor belt

On 6 August 2020, I had a bone marrow biopsy, the gold standard for confirming the diagnosis. The date is Kylie's birthday and, coincidentally, Hiroshima Day – the day the American military dropped the first atomic bomb – which was a very significant day in my life for a few reasons.

Advised to take the public patient pathway in my local hospital, I was allocated to a haematologist who is a skilled researcher and medical expert but not a good communicator. At our first meeting, Chris and I were in shock. The feelings of disbelief and grief were new to me, and I felt numb.

I ask others, 'What was I like?' The feedback is alarming and feels true. Apparently, I was confused and very angry, felt 'bitten on the bum', deceived by my body, frightened of the treatment, distrustful of the pharmacology, powerless and reliant on a doctor who refused to communicate with me. I felt that I was on my path to death, and I was scared. Friends were unaccustomed to seeing me frightened, lacking confidence and 'snappy'.

I was given the haematologist's prognosis whether I wanted it or not. I didn't want to be told how long my doctor thought I'd live. I am unique and I have never fitted into the bell curve so why would that be true now? If his 'best guess' is true, I hope to die with dignity. To live until I say goodbye, with laughter out measuring tears.

I remembered a quote from Gail O'Brien's book about medical predictions: 'Well, that's all bullshit and you know it,' a brain surgeon colleague told Chris O'Brien. 'Patients decide how long they will live, you know that. Doctors don't decide how long patients have. We've both made that mistake.'

The 'best guess' rule is not a death sentence. Medicine is not absolute. Even the best scan is only an indication of what is happening inside our bodies. The best drugs only work well when they do; some of us will not comply with even the best of research predictions; some of us will sleep well with minute doses of anaesthetic, while others need to be knocked out cold, and still they tell tales of the surgical procedure they 'witnessed'.

Tubi offered wise words: 'Mum, myeloma just took a shot across your bow.' Friends have called it a 'twist in the path' or a 'fork in the road'. I didn't name my feelings at the time or even remember them, there were no words to articulate them. From that winter night in July until now, I am just surviving. I have cancer.

The events of the first three months settled on my consciousness like a burning log; sometimes there was a bright clean flame, tricky but hopeful, and at other times there was smouldering fear and hopelessness. I comprehended most of the medical language and I understood monoclonal antibodies, because our PhD students made them in the research lab 20 years ago.

From the first meeting with the haematology oncologist, I knew he was not the doctor for me. When we met (after enduring a long meeting with his registrar), I told him that I was a scientist, and I would understand my situation in medical terms. Could he please explain it to me? This powerful, shy man spoke to his computer screen and his nurse in riddles. Not once did he look directly at me. Was I actually experiencing this non-conversation about my life-or-death situation?

What I took from the 'riddles' was that I was very sick, and I must start immunomodulatory therapy as soon as possible. What I heard was that I was lucky because this gold standard treatment was newly approved by the TGA and would be free. I didn't feel lucky.

After we left the meeting, I asked Chris what his notes said (Chris recorded our medical consultations as I had gone selectively deaf with anxiety and fear) he replied, 'That guy doesn't like giving bad news.'

## Dreaded side effects

Over the next week, I started a triple-drug therapy designed to last for six months or less. Gosh, that felt like forever, yet in retrospect, it actually flew past! I received a subcutaneous injection in my abdominal fat once a week and two other drugs taken orally.

The standard dose combination hit me hard initially and I had a severe allergic reaction. My skin fell off! Within hours I couldn't do any normal bodily chores like shower myself and brushing my teeth was exhausting.

I went to the oncology outpatients and my haematologist reviewed me, gave me drugs to lessen the side effects of treatment and topped me up with a saline drip. My skin settled down then my throat started up. I returned to oncology outpatients and was told I had a herpes infection of my oesophagus, from my tonsils to my stomach. My mouth became a burning inferno. That was why I couldn't swallow anything, not even water. I lost 10 kgs in 10 days – the most frightening part of the long saga. I couldn't stop the weight loss. I vowed never to diet again if I survived that torture.

There is nothing like chemotherapy to stop you in your tracks. When you can get your mind off your physical suffering, like how to drink water when you have herpes ulcers from the back of your throat to your stomach! There is always the emotional torture. 'What if I die of this disease?' 'Should I buy new pyjamas or risk buying 'going out' clothes?' 'Should I bother going to the dentist if I'm going to die anyway?' There is too much time to think as you spend your days moving from the bed to the couch and back again as the aches and pains of your aging bones take charge of your mind.

But wait, there's more – I then suffered the worst urinary tract infection (UTI) ever.

I want to tell every emergency department doctor and nurse that they have to act quickly and prescribe an antibiotic ASAP because by the time folk (like me) turn up at the hospital with a UTI, they have endured hours of pain and suffering, hoping the gallons of water they drink will ease the suffering. That person in the ER cubicle is in agony. This is not deadly, but it certainly feels like torture. Do you hear me?

## An exasperated patient

During treatment, my days were spent sleeping in our bed or on the lounge, lifting my head to eat very little and going back to mindless TV or sleep. Each day, Chris showered me, even when I couldn't stand up, oiled my skin with fabulous oil that my children bought me and dressed me in clothes that I could tolerate against my skin. I was an invalid, and I was fortunate to have a loving and gentle man nursing me.

Each week we went to the hospital and the nurse on duty that day asked me about any side effects of treatment, she then reported to the registrar on duty who offered me advice – through the nurse, rarely the same nurse each time and it was never the doctor dispensing the advice. This was a very strange procedure. Why didn't anyone in the system attempt to develop a human relationship with me? No doctor spoke to me directly about my medical challenges.

The culture of cancer treatment is like any organisation – it depends on the leader. I have visited cancer centres in Scotland, Portland, Seattle, Sydney and Melbourne and now Canberra. I have seen the best and the worst of it. Keeping cancer patients at arm's length isn't a guarantee that you won't be diagnosed with cancer yourself, or that your heart won't break when others die or suffer. At QFL, we would say that it is okay for your heart to break because when it heals it grows bigger with scar tissue. Petrea King says, 'If you didn't want suffering, you should have gone to another planet; planet earth is about suffering.'

On a subsequent visit to the haematologist, he advised me not to take any supplements while I was undergoing treatment, and I agreed. I did commission a firm to do my genomic testing and I asked him to send a sample to the lab I had chosen. It took a lot of pressure from the pathologist at the genomics lab for my haematologist to finally release the sample of my bone marrow. It was a poor specimen, barely useable and the haematologist's team were very uncooperative.

The family and I were actually managing very well. We knew the rhythm of the weekly cycle. There was a build-up of side effects over the first two days after the injection and then a slow recovery until we returned for another injection the next week. Would it ever end? Or would I die? Each month or two I met with the specialist and that was the worst part of the cycle. A few days before the appointment I would start rehearsing my introductory words: 'Good afternoon, how am I going?' or, 'I'm feeling more and more anxious about my treatment, and I'd like to understand what is happening to me medically,' or, 'When is my next PET scan scheduled?' or, 'I'd like to know your plan for me?'

By the time I sat in front of him, I was a 72-year-old, grey-haired lady who felt trivialised and brainless. As our session ended, I would be ushered out without a conversation. I remember getting angry with Chris because he didn't 'stick up' for me in the meeting with the haematologist. What did I want him to do for me? I didn't know. I just needed to get my brain out of the 'chemo fog' and regain a sense of control over this life-limiting situation.

In April, I was scheduled to have a second bone marrow biopsy. I told the genomic testing lab and they asked for a small sample to be collected for them. On the day of the procedure, I asked the registrar for the sample and she rang the haematologist, who refused to let her put some of my bone marrow into fixative for the genomics pathologist. I was torn between letting the procedure go ahead and stopping it. I decided to have the biopsy (a very painful test) and deal with the injustice later. The bone marrow showed that I was in a 'very good partial remission' (VGPR) and eventually the genomics lab got a small sample but in the wrong fixative, so it was again useless. If I ever have another bone marrow biopsy, the genomics lab has promised to process it for free.

In May, the injections stopped, and I started to reduce one of the drugs that scared me the most. In fact, I didn't want to take it, from the very first pill. I knew that it was extremely toxic, it stopped the production of my own adrenalin by replacing it. The specialist began the process and dropped the dose from 20-12 mgs and in desperation, due to side effects, I dropped it to 8mgs. Side effects included extreme bloating, 6-12 hours of incontinence on the day I took the drug, red flushed face, sleeplessness for three nights after I took the tablet and finally, by mid-May 2021, I had brown smudges before my eyes. The GP and the optometrist were wonderfully supportive medically, however I still struggle with my eyes most days. The drop to 8 mgs helped take away the smudges but I still felt terrible most of the time.

It will take my body a long time to recover from 13 months of treatment with this particular drug alone.

### Taking back some control

I arranged to see the hospital psychologist and assessed my options for a different haematologist. I had completed a research survey for Myeloma Australia, based in Melbourne, so felt comfortable talking with them about my situation. They suggested a Canberra-based doctor in their research group who I could see in three days' time. She was a great communicator and Chris and I had tears in our eyes during the consultation as we finally felt 'heard'. By the end of June, I was seeing my naturopath and taking supplements. At the next visit, I showed the new haematologist what natural products I was taking, as I had advised clients to do for years (international best practice from

Integrative Oncology research). The response was, 'They are all fine, please add a probiotic!' Immediately she told me to STOP the drug that was giving me all the eye problems. Sadly, in the midst of my enthusiasm, I stopped the 8 mgs dose straight away when I should have eased myself off it. I had withdrawal problems and even my delight at being off the drug didn't stop me feeling terrible for a couple of weeks.

I had to become a private patient in order to see another haematologist, and I am still not sure what that will mean in the long term.

## What now?

I have reservations about where I am up to now, only time will tell. If it works out, then I will have found the right doctor for me. If not, I will keep looking. Life is precious and quality of life is priceless. I was reliant on the grumpy haematologist, who thought so differently from me, for over a year. He held my medical cancer history in his head and on his computer, maybe I was even a number in one of the drug trials he was running? Even though I have taken back some control, I feel a bit 'rudderless' right now.

Over the years at QFL and in my clinic, I had advised folk to find the right doctor for them, never knowing just what I was asking of them. I certainly know now. Changing haematologists sounds easy, but it really wasn't. I wish I had shown more empathy in those conversations. It is a terrible thing to ask folk to do, without doctor number one I was alone in my medical file. How very difficult it is to change doctors when it is your life that is hanging in the balance.

Today, I was reminded about the question, 'How are you, really?' especially when it is followed by a deep long look into your face. 'Well… I don't know. I don't know who I am or where I'm headed.' Rarely do I think about dying or what lies between now and death. I am chugging through each day much like everyone else…eating my baked beans on toast on cold days and walking in the sunshine and rain.

I have watched and listened to many people make life and death decisions and now it's my turn. I have all the knowledge in my head from my years at QFL, science from the lab days and my spiritual journey up until now. What decisions I make will be one by one, one day at a time. Each confrontation with a medical assessment team brings apprehension and relief. Every pain is a reminder that I have cancer. The spectre of recurrence is always sitting on my left shoulder. I hope I will be on planet earth for as long as it takes to finish what needs my presence to complete.

# 11.

# Reflections

You now know so much about me: my achievements, missteps and the ups and downs of passionately (and stubbornly) following a dream. Was I successful? Only time will tell whether I 'tossed my pearls before swine' in my OM journey.

Eleven is a number that brings a rueful smile to my face because of the YouTube clip *Two Scotsmen in a voice activated lift*. Why? In the joke, their words fall on deaf ears. The frustrated travellers try everything – speaking another language, shouting louder, 'swearing', but nothing changes. The lift doesn't move, and the 11th floor remains out of reach. Twenty years of promoting and teaching oncology massage is my parallel experience and I'm still jumping up and down in the 'lift of life' with my book in hand. Does anyone hear?

> When I mention OM, some health professionals say, 'I've never heard of it.' I was struggling with chemotherapy, with an aching

> back, and the advice the RN gave me was to 'have a remedial massage'. Quite apart from my compromised immune system, I have a compression fracture of my 12th vertebra, so... no. Sometimes bad advice is worse than no advice at all.

For over 20 years, I have been spreading the 'good news,' with real-life stories and research of amazing OM achievements. There are thousands of therapists working with tens of thousands of clients around the world, yet OM remains a mystery to most of the general public. Those whose lives have been touched by a cancer diagnosis have only a 30 per cent chance of asking about OM and less than a 10 per cent chance of receiving an OM. This is despite research showing that pain and anxiety are lowered by well over 50 per cent when OM is given by a trained OM therapist. Why is this so? Could it be that OM is trapped in the abyss that exists in Australia between medicine and complementary therapies? An entrenched belief system based on fear and misunderstanding, which is like the children's game of Chinese whispers in many cases. The players don't have bad intent; it's just that the story is not relayed accurately.

During immunomodulatory therapy, I was yearning for an OM but ironically, I couldn't get in to see a qualified OM therapist. Eventually, when my mind could cope, I saw a local remedial therapist whom I coached as she massaged me. This skilled therapist has never been taught any science of cancer, how cancer treatment affects the body or the role of the relaxation response in healing. She was far too young to have any knowledge of the convalescent hospitals of my youth or the work of Dr Herbert Benson. Fortunately for me, she understood what I needed, and I settled into deep relaxation.

Do we need more OM-trained therapists in Australia? Yes, we do!

## What am I most proud of?

My heart bursts with pride when I think about the clients I massaged. The brave folk who allowed me to 'work things out' as I went along – the lymphedema softened, the pain and anxiety were relieved and the fear of abandonment was suspended while I worked.

I feel pride when I think of the heartfelt feelings and passion that have driven me on over the years and do still. Tenacity, I guess, and pigheadedness – a double-edged sword.

And then there were moments when the world told me I had made a difference.

Over the years, I have chosen to attend only a few funerals. I remember them all. In one eulogy, the husband spoke about the last massage I gave his dying wife. He told the congregation that I changed everything.

> It was a very cold winter night on a remote farm. The lounge room was very draughty and the fire was devouring wood quickly. The youngish mum was cold and frightened, unable to leave her recliner without help, as her legs were twice their normal size. I set about tucking in her blankets, popping a beanie on her head and offering her a drink of warm water. I did the OM leg massage over her pyjama pants for 15 minutes on each leg. She fell fast asleep. I didn't know until the eulogy that the ambulance came an hour later and took her to the hospice, where she died. He said 'The peace I found when I came home that last night was unforgettable. I called the ambulance. I can never thank Eleanor enough for her kindness.'

Yes, I am most proud of the 'work' and my worth. The patients I have been privileged to touch and massage. Leaving every oncology massage knowing I had made a difference.

> '*Worth is when we cry for people. Crying matters. When I cry with tears for other people, I know the goodness inside me.*'
> (Yanyuwa people)

This is the perfect place to 'hoist the flag', hold our heads high and raise awareness of OM therapists and teachers, office staff, industry associations and industry magazines. Without their support over the past 20-plus years, I would never have kept going. Words alone cannot tell the story of the calibre of women and men, wonderful therapists, who joined me. I am deeply proud of the people drawn to OM. Humility and inclusiveness, compassion and passion, persistence and perseverance. We have all experienced judgement, criticism and betrayal, and yet we have kept going. I haven't named every therapist and teacher and I know who I have referred to, and so do they. May we all remember what we have achieved in our working life as OM therapists and be proud.

## What would I say to my younger self?

Wake up sooner, little Eleanor.

That is probably a bit harsh as everything I learned over all the years of science, military life, marriage and massage gave me the background to understand bodies, people and life choices in general, but it wasn't enough.

I'd tell her to learn about her inner demons sooner. What old beliefs about yourself are driving your self-talk, fears and inner thinking?

Moving out of science was when my journey of self-discovery began in earnest, and I was 50! The path to massaging folk with cancer was like a superhighway, and it was the only way I could remain true to myself.

I would tell my younger self not to hide behind the marriage, the demands of motherhood, moving house often and a plethora of excuses I gave myself to 'linger' on the path of life. Procrastination robbed me of chances to learn more, do more, and contribute more to the wellbeing of others.

## What did I learn about myself?

My first step in learning about myself was at QFL. Petrea King touched my heart from the minute we met. She heard me, on many levels. She accepted me 'warts and all' and because of the 'warts', in spite of myself, she allowed me to grow and experience the ME that was locked inside. I was desperately trying to get things right for everyone else. My experience gave me a place where I could be myself. Love on legs!

I learned that I'm a really nice person. That I'm smart (even if dyslexia robbed me of spelling confidence) and passionate about bringing compassion and comfort to people in need. I learned that I make good decisions and follow through. I laugh a lot at myself and never at others. At 73 years old, I like who I am. I'm brave and naïve, not stupid. I am either self-sacrificing or determined and ambitious. I'm complex and that's okay.

## What was the hardest part?

The hardest parts of my journey with OM have been the business side of things and what others projected onto me as my 'intent'. Almost without exception, folk in business thought I was teaching OM for the money. In reality, I have not earned enough to pay tax since 2000. In my utopian world, I would be paid fairly for my client work, my teaching and my counselling skills. The community and/or government would fund IO (Integrative Oncology) for every person with cancer. If we could create a fee scale that made OM affordable for everyone, we could set up massage services, delivered by well-trained therapists, in every aged care facility and medical service in our 'lucky country'.

What if a massage department provided massage to medical staff at the time of injury in the workplace, providing compassionate care for every nurse's back injury? Taking as good care of staff as hospitals do of patients? What IF?

It was heartbreaking to have 'empty pockets' when a little money (nothing like pharmaceutical industry funding) could have opened doors to OM that remain closed to this day. The Sydney hospital massage training program ended because the hospital could not find money to keep it going even when it was very successful. Why? Because medical principles are applied to massage work. They didn't understand at all, they just thought they did. The pictures in the foyer were worth more than it would have taken to develop an OM service in that particular hospital.

On reflection, I had my head in the sand when it came to running a business. I never made the time to learn how to read a balance sheet accurately. I could get the gist of things, the bottom line, but nothing more. I thought that was enough, but it wasn't. I never got into debt or was unable to pay bills. We all worked long hours for very little money. Bless their hearts, Kylie and the first Board tried to compensate me for all the early work I had done to establish OMT, and I am grateful for the partial remuneration I was able to receive as a result.

I did a semester of sociology (remember I told you that my teeth were clenched for six months?), however I didn't apply the global behaviour of money and business to my 'little' business and that is what kept it 'little'. If I had taken out a loan when Kylie was in full swing, she would have had a better chance of success in building a sustainable training organisation, large enough to meet the current needs.

Eventually, there were too many folk talking up another agenda, with conflicting priorities, and I lacked the business skills to identify what was needed. I thought I could rely on the system, and it let me down. Christine Scott and Tammy Boatman at Austin Health were 'moved on' not long after they had achieved industry awards and glowing recognition. The head of cancer services and radiation oncology (my strongest advocates) at The Austin disappeared too. I told everyone that there were financial challenges with OM services in hospitals. Hospitals have to pay for them, insurance companies won't and the government ministers were too busy keeping the 'ship afloat' to understand what the CM and IO services were offering the oncology programs. Without philanthropy, OM services will remain limited to the wealthy.

## What could happen in the health system to make integrative care more sustainable?

In 2001, I thought it was important to develop an accredited training program that met all the same government standards as medically trained professions, qualifications like paramedics and dental technicians. All the OM teachers did 'train the trainer' certificates and upgraded them as the ASQA guidelines demanded. I thought that research would lead to sustainability, as it did in Scotland. Through the Iris Foundation scoping study and financial support from the Iris Foundation, Gayle has created a strong OM workforce across the whole of Scotland. Without a similar level of support from a charity, philanthropist or our Cancer Council, this was just not possible in Australia.

An email arrived today from a colleague, a PhD student in Melbourne who is on the development team at the largest cancer hospital in Australia:

> *For my part, I am still plugging away, have completed all the course work for the doctorate and now in the stage of serious study design and ethics approval. I am already grey headed, but*

> *I might just make it! I hope more than anything else to inspire others. 'Bottom up' advocacy from consumers is important but we need the wherewithal to generate 'top down' collaboration as well, as you well know.'*

There are many reasons why integrative care for cancer patients walks a fine line in our culture and our medical system. Clients know our worth, but they are sick. When they get better, we are part of the 'bad old days'. Family members know our worth during the illness and treatment or in the last days of life – they even talk about us in the eulogy, but we remain part of one of the saddest events that life can dish up. Again, we are forgotten. Friends and family give gift vouchers to folk with cancer for a facial, spa treatment or massage but rarely oncology massage. Even the person with cancer doesn't want to see their name alongside the word oncology. After the last two years of hosting multiple myeloma in my body, I don't want my name linked to the words 'cancer' or 'oncology' if I can avoid it.

If our oncologists and GPs embraced IO and OM by writing a referral for a series of massages, an assessment with an exercise physiologist and a nutritionist, and information about cancer support groups in their suburb, then IO would be in full swing.

I have met only a handful of medical staff in my treatment for myeloma, but not one has engaged with me – the being, the scientist, the mother, the wife, the sister, the friend or, God forbid, the massage professional! They have infused me, bone marrow-ed me, injected me, taken my vitals, yet almost two years into treatment, there isn't one person who knows my name without my file. Not even the oncologist who saved my life. Thank God for my GP.

Integrating OM into our current medical model wasn't about science. Science wasn't the answer, and top-notch research out of MSKCC wasn't enough to even spark curiosity. Remember the young doctors in the palliative care ward at the Austin on that very first day we took OM into that sacred space? They knew the worth of OM – hope springs eternal.

Over the years, two conversations developed around me: 'Why do you want to work with people who have cancer and are (most likely) dying?' and, 'You have to write a book.'

I have (mostly) stopped working with folk on the edge of life and here I am writing my book.

## A final reflection

I think I have said what I want to say about myself, my work and our medical system. When folk are on a path that most likely leads to the end of their life, they don't want platitudes or coffin eyes. They need truth, reality and compassion in order to celebrate a life well lived and to embrace forgiveness of themselves and others.

What has changed me the most in my life is my work as an OM therapist. I heard the truth about myself, from within myself and from compassionate others. That 'truth' (as it was at the time) gave me direction and challenge. We are all a work in progress until our last breath and we can see it as an adventure or as a burden.

The reality is that we all have to die. Can I meet this reality with wisdom and peace? John Coleman gave me a little book years ago called *When I Love Myself Enough*, that encourages me to 'let myself off the hook', let go of my internal 'shoulds' and forgive myself for a lifetime of being human.

*Compassion* led me to OM and is still my driving force. Compassion is the secret ingredient of all safe touch – from your lover, your friend, your health professional and your massage therapist. Compassion for yourself and others. Once you realise that everyone has a story of challenge, grief, struggle and want, you can open your heart without fear. Every client I have been privileged to touch (massage) has shared some of their life story verbally and silently through the physical changes I feel. Intimacy is inevitable when compassionate touch connects with suffering.

Every OM massage therapist brings compassion with them to work every day in the face of continued resistance, distrust and unspoken demands of the medical community. I take my hat off to each and every one of them and send them my deepest gratitude for their dedication and service.

# 12.

# How Can We Live Our Best Lives?

It is fitting that this last chapter goes beyond my reflections and gives the reader some practical information based on what I have learned and try to apply in my life.

In Chapter 2, I talked about the vital role of our immune system in maintaining our health. So, it is really important to identify and manage the things in life that worry our immune system and increase the risk that things can go wrong. Principally, these are challenges like relentless emotional stress (e.g. divorce, grief, family breakdown), chemical stressors (e.g. everyday exposure to toxic fumes that are absorbed through our skin and nostrils) and poor nutrition from an ever-changing food chain.

How do we support our immune system to keep doing what it does best: protecting us from ill health and disease? We cannot remove all the challenges of life. But we can minimise the stresses on our mind and body and find ways to reduce the impact of unavoidable stress.

## Listen to our bodies

When a diagnosis comes as a surprise, it might feel that even a heart attack comes out of the blue. I often hear clients say that they were 'never sick a day in their life' until they were diagnosed with advanced cancer. We have so many ways of tricking our mind and body into 'soldiering on' that we don't notice the many and varied messages we do get. Our bodies give us subtle messages all the time like fatigue, constipation and 'dire-rear', loss of appetite, overeating or unexplained weight loss.

I think we live from the eyebrows up! Then a disease stops us in our tracks, and we begin to notice our fatigue, thirst, broken sleep patterns and hurtful relationships. We can support our healing by addressing these issues. This is the basis of naturopathy, homeopathy and other complementary medicine (CM) therapies.

## Think about toxins

> The first part of my life was pretty toxin-free except for DDT and nuclear fallout from Maralinga! But I shudder to think of how many toxic substances went into my body when I worked in cytology. We scientists were very 'gung-ho'. In 1967, I was setting up the first white cell counting machine in haematology, and I shot the mercury in the counter-balance out onto the floor. I gathered the little pellets of mercury into my hand and popped them into a petri dish. My boss was more worried about possible damage to my new engagement ring than my exposure to the highly toxic substance!

Did you know that there are at least 100,000 chemicals on the planet that were not here 50 years ago? I know that many wonderful things in my life have evolved from developments in the chemical and pharmaceutical industries. However, there are 42 neurotoxins in the breast milk of Inuit women that are also in the breast milk of women in California. There is not a woman on the planet who can offer her child neurotoxin-free breast milk.

It is said that toxins don't cause cancer. Of course, they do. I grew neurons in tissue culture and if I got one ingredient slightly out, too much or too little in a microscopic amount, the neurons died. If I cleaned the equipment with the wrong detergent or didn't rinse it thoroughly enough, the neurons died. I know that chemicals in our bodies matter to our cells and to the enzyme pathways that convert food to support life.

We live on a toxic planet, and we need to do everything we can to minimise the stress on our bodies caused by the constant need to neutralise chemicals that were never meant to be there. Think about the cleaning products you use, the chemicals you apply in the garden – there are great alternatives out there that will work well and be better for you and our planet.

> Next time you have a massage, ask what oil or cream the practitioner is using on your body. If it is not a certified organic, petroleum-free product, get off the table and find another massage therapist!

## Eat SLOW food

We can do a lot to support our bodies, especially by putting effort and thought into what we eat. It is not about a special diet or drinking juice with grass in it. Healthy eating is about seasonal, local, organic and whole: SLOW food.

Zach Bush MD is a physician specialising in internal medicine, endocrinology and hospice care with a focus on the microbiome (the bacteria in our intestines) as it relates to health and disease. Zach talks about the health of the soil and our farming practices as they relate to emerging diseases. Zach's website is worth a look (zachbushmd.com). It is in cartoon style, so the information can be easily understood by all ages.

If you can afford organic food from a respected retailer, that is a great place to start. If that is not possible, remember two rules when choosing fruit and vegetables from your local supermarket: select produce from the top of the stack and buy what is in season. If you can buy local produce with very low food miles, that is a bonus.

> I grew up on homegrown, chemical-free vegetables. Meat carcasses were delivered to the local butcher and prepared for sale in his shop, and bread and milk arrived on our doorstep every morning. In our home, Chris and I have always eaten meals together, with our children when they were growing up. Our table was a fun, lively, convivial place to be most of the time, shared by family and friends. We prepared whole food, even when we were in the busiest years, both working full time with three children. It was not easy, but I believe it was important to the health of us all.

In my work with folk with cancer, I have witnessed some healthy diets and some very unusual diets. Some seem to improve health and others have increased stress so much that the diet is totally robbing the sick person of their quality of life.

If you don't like juice, don't drink it! Eat your food slowly, enjoy the flavours and invite healing in with every mouthful.

Diet and exercise advice for cancer patients is complex and often delivered as fleeting remarks. I'd love to see patients given heartfelt lectures by nurses or, better still, oncologists. The importance of regular exercise and a healthy gut is downplayed by many specialists. Encouragingly, in recent times, medical scientists have explored the human biome (bacteria in our small and large intestine that facilitate digestion and balance our pH) so we are witnessing a positive shift in the medical community's attitude towards diet. Exercise during chemotherapy treatment is advertised widely in cancer treatment units, along with meditation and yoga. As the 'fundamentals' of treatment and cancer care change quickly in today's world, it is not always easy for patients to do things that will help.

> As I struggled through the early days of cancer treatment, the last thing I felt like doing was exercising or eating salad. I spent six months going from my bed to the couch via the shower then back to bed again. Eventually, I walked to a neighbour's house and lay on the couch while we chatted. By the end of the first year, my legs were like jelly, my tummy slack and round and my morale very low. The Zoom lectures from Myeloma Australia were all about treatment options, exercise and not getting 'fat'. I really struggled to maintain my natural optimism and avoid feeling like a failure. Finally, I remembered to tell myself, 'You are sick, Eleanor. Rest, eat sooky food and let yourself off the hook. Praise all your healthy cells and ask the cancer cells to leave now. Plan a return to exercise and a more structured diet when your body says yes.'

## Live our best lives

Caryle Hirshberg and Mark Barasch published a fantastic book in 1995 based on their study of 6,000 people who were diagnosed with cancer and told they had three to six months to live.[20] They all went on to live well and disease-free, long beyond their 'allotted' time. These folk had a spontaneous remission, as Petrea King did when she was 32 years old. Petrea also investigated the qualities found in people who flourish and through her work, the 4Cs were born: Regain Control, Commitment to Living, Sense of Challenge and Sense of Connection.[21] For over 30 years, she has used these four qualities of resilience and peace of mind to underpin her workshops for the QFL Foundation. The 4Cs explain how the essence of who we are determines how we manage a life-limiting diagnosis and how who we are changes throughout life. We are not a victim of our genes; we are dynamic fluid beings. Our job is to find the environment in which healing can happen.

> I sat beside Petrea for almost nine years, sharing her week-long program with the participants as they figured themselves out. Who am I, now that I have a life-limiting disease? I often asked, 'What stands between you and peace today?' It was often the job, the spouse, the boss, the bank balance or the pain. By the end of the week, we saw the result of the relaxation response and Petrea's 4Cs. It felt like a sense of hope. Not a hope that they wouldn't die – a hope that they would live well today.

What we think and feel changes our biology moment by moment. Consequently, fear and powerlessness initiate a toxic bunch of chemicals. Being 'real' matters – it's not about being positive and happy all the time. Saying what you are feeling matters. Getting up

---

[20] Caryle Hirshberg & Marc Ian Barasch (1995) *Remarkable recovery: what extraordinary healings tell us about getting well and staying well.* New York: Riverhead Books.
[21] https://questforlife.org.au/toolkit/toolkit-for-adults/#6

to date with your past by understanding what happened. Forgiveness liberates you from the sea of chemicals attached to your fears, regrets and self-judgements. Your life matters first.

Could it be that it is the intensity of a cancer diagnosis and treatment that stops us in our tracks? That gives us space to think and get up to date with our relationship with ourselves? Science tells us that if the cell surface receptors change and adapt, if we can potentiate our cells with anandamide, clean up the interstitial sea by removing toxins from our environment, eat organic SLOW food and deeply connect with our emotions, maybe the cell science of epigenetics can be shown to be right? Maybe we can bring hope to healing.

> I chose to have chemotherapy when I was diagnosed with myeloma in multiple bones throughout my body. My thinking was that this would buy me time to put my belief system into action. I believe that cancer treatment is not a competition between medical science and natural healing principles, it is a smorgasbord, and our job is to listen to advice, and choose from the 'feast'. We need to learn to listen to our intuition, our inner tutor. We don't get it right every time, or even most of the time, but we do get better at listening to ourselves.
>
> I have been exposed to many toxic chemicals over the years and I have eaten well, rested and relaxed when time permitted and developed my relationships when I could, and yet I still got cancer. There is no single way to avoid illness on planet earth, if there were we would be taught how to in preschool.
>
> Avoid feelings of blame and shame. Endeavour to see every fork in the road as an adventure and don't internalise your experience of cancer as a 'battle'. Nobody needs a fight inside their own body. We could develop a sense of curiosity and

exploration of our new normal now that we have cancer. I'm working on me!

# About the Author

Eleanor entered Sydney Technical College in 1966 where she studied Medical Technology. Haematology and the Blood Bank at St Vincent's Hospital laid the foundation for a 30-year career in Pathology and Medical Research. She specialised in cytology – diagnosing cancer by light microscopy.

For ten years Eleanor was the technical manager of a developmental neuroscience research laboratory at the John Curtin School of Medical Research at the Australian National University in Canberra. It was during this time Eleanor developed an intimate understanding of neurons, tissues culture, monoclonal antibodies, in-situ hybridization and collaborative research.

At age 50, in 1998, Eleanor went to massage school and on completion of a Diploma of Remedial Massage and Bowen therapy she wrote the first ten-week pathology course for massage schools in Canberra. This was a first for Australia.

Eleanor went on to work with Petrea King at Quest for Life Centre, facilitating residential cancer programs and developing specialised OM training for massage therapists. She developed a nationally consistent training program and trained skilled therapists to deliver the program across Australia.

Eleanor taught massage students around Australia and in New Zealand, Germany and Hong Kong. In 2016 she visited Spain and developed training opportunities with the prestigious ISMET Massage School in Barcelona. Eleanor also taught in The Netherlands.

Eleanor established the first two in-hospital training programs in Australia, in 2009 at the Sydney Adventist Hospital, Sydney and in 2012 at the Olivia Newton John Cancer, Research and Wellness Centre, The Austin Hospital, Melbourne which continues today.

Over the past 22 years, Eleanor has published her opinions in professional journals and magazines. In 2015 Eleanor embarked on research with Western Sydney University, National Institute of Complementary Medicine and results were published in November 2017.

OMG began in 2017 teaching OM in Spanish and English. The company is a consultancy designed to take oncology massage around the world, based on our Australian experience since 2000.

Eleanor lives in Canberra, ACT, with her husband, Chris, and grown family nearby. One day she may retire.

www.oncologymassageglobal.com.au

**'Oncology Massage Success Blueprint'**
Download today from OMG website and build your confidence.
Contact: info@oncologymassageglobal.com.au
for more information.

# Acronyms and Abbreviations

| | |
|---|---|
| ANPA | Australian Naturopathic Practitioners' Association |
| ARCCIM | Australian Research Centre in Complementary and Integrative Medicine |
| ASQA | Australian Skills Quality Authority |
| ATMS | Australian Traditional Medicine Society |
| BAA | Bowen Association of Australia |
| BT | Bowen therapy |
| BTFA | Bowen Therapy Federation of Australia |
| COSA | Clinical Oncology Society of Australia |
| CM | Complementary medicine |
| DON | Director of Nursing |
| DVT | Deep vein thrombosis |
| FNA | Fine needle aspiration |
| ICU | Intensive Care Unit |
| IO | Integrative Oncology |
| ISBT | International Society of Bowen |
| ISMET | Instituto Superior de Medicinas Tradicionales (Spain). |
| JCSMR | John Curtin School of Medical Research (Canberra) |
| MC&M | Massage, Cancer & More |
| MSKCC | Memorial Sloan Kettering Cancer Centre (New York) |

| | |
|---|---|
| NSWCI | NSW Cancer Institute |
| NUM | Nurse Unit Manager |
| OM | Oncology massage |
| OMG | Oncology Massage Global |
| OML | Oncology Massage Limited |
| OMT | Oncology Massage Training |
| ONJCW&RC | Olivia Newton John Cancer Wellness & Research Centre |
| PPE | Personal protective equipment |
| PNG | Papua New Guinea |
| QFL | Quest for Life Centre (Bundanoon, NSW) |
| RTO | Registered Training Organisation |
| SIO | Society for Integrative Oncology (US) |
| S4OM | Society for Oncology Massage (US) |
| TCM | Traditional Chinese Medicine |
| UK | United Kingdom |
| US | United States |
| UTS | University of Technology Sydney |
| WSU | Western Sydney University |

# Further Reading

**Oncology Massage**

Janet Penny and Rebecca L Sturgeon (2021) *Oncology Massage: an integrative approach to cancer care*. London: Handspring Publishing Ltd.

Gayle MacDonald (1999). *Medicine Hands: Massage Therapy for People with Cancer*. Scotland: Findhorn Press. 877 390 4425.

Gayle MacDonald (2004). *Massage for the Hospital Patient and Medically Frail Client*. Philadelphia: Lippincott Williams & Wilkins.

Tracy Walton (2020) *Medical Conditions and Massage Therapy: A Decision Tree Approach*. US: Jones & Bartlett Learning.

**Anatomy and Body Mind Science**

Herbert Benson (2000) *The Relaxation Response*. US: HarperCollins.

John Coleman (2020) *Rethinking Parkinson's Disease*. AU: New Holland Publishers.

Phyllis K Davis (1999) *The Power of Touch*. US: Hay House.

Gabor Mate (2019) *When the Body Says No: The Cost of Hidden Stress*. AU: Scribe.

Thomas W Myers (2020) *Anatomy Trains: Myofascial Meridians for Manual and Movement Therapists*. UK: Elsevier.

Thomas W Myers and James Earls (2017) *Fascial Release for Structural Balance*. UK: Lotus Publishing.

Candace B Pert (1997). *Molecules of Emotion: The Science Behind Mind Body Medicine*. Simon and Schuster: US.

**Inspirational**

Brene Brown (2018) *Dare to Lead*. UK: Random House.

Petrea King (2005) *Your Life Matters: The Power of Living Now*. AU: Random House.

Ngaanyatjarra Pitantjatjara Yankunytjatjara Women's Council Aboriginal Corporation (2013) *Traditional Healers of Central Australia: Ngangkari*. Australia: Magabala Books.

Juliette O'Brien (2016) *This is Gail: Life with and after Chris O'Brien*. Australia: Harper Collins.

Rachael Naomi Remen (2021) *Kitchen Table Wisdom*. UK: Pan Macmillan.

# Acknowledgements

As a self-confessed details person when telling a story, I could start with gratitude for the doctor who delivered me and finish with my new neighbour who brought us soup on the first night in our new house... but I won't.

I feel gratitude for my whole life, all the folk who loved and moulded me, even those who found fault and told me so!

The clients who trusted me with their fragile bodies; the colleagues who listened to me while I talked my ideas into action; the scientists and supervisors who shared insights, explaining until I understood; my massage teachers who told me I had 'good hands'; and my family and friends who shared the rollercoaster of life with me and still do.

This book requires special thanks for the tireless work of Elizabeth Hall. This book could not have been written, certainly not finished, without Elizabeth. Her unique talent with words, her encouraging manner and her heart overflowing with compassion for humanity guided me through the soul-searching journey that telling my story became. I had no idea what I was asking when we began. I know now.

The team at Ultimate 48Hour Author provided a framework for me to 'see' possibilities and creative pathways to our finished product.

I have acknowledged others in my manuscript and dedication and the last 'thank you' is for my husband Chris. He inspired *Touching Cancer*, financed my vision and holds me in safe arms as I release my 'pearls of wisdom'.

One lifetime is too short to share with Chris. Can we have another one?

Love and 'hugs a plenty' to all who read *Touching Cancer*, you have been touched by the suffering of life and a little kind touch could be a blessing.

Eleanor

# Notes

# TOUCHING CANCER

# Notes

www.ingramcontent.com/pod-product-compliance
Lightning Source LLC
Chambersburg PA
CBHW030036100526
44590CB00011B/225